# TANTRA YONI MASSAGE THE DANCE OF ECSTASY

*A Step-by-Step Guide to the Art of Tantric Massages, for Perfect Touches and the Awakening of Your Kundalini Energy Through Illustrated Techniques*

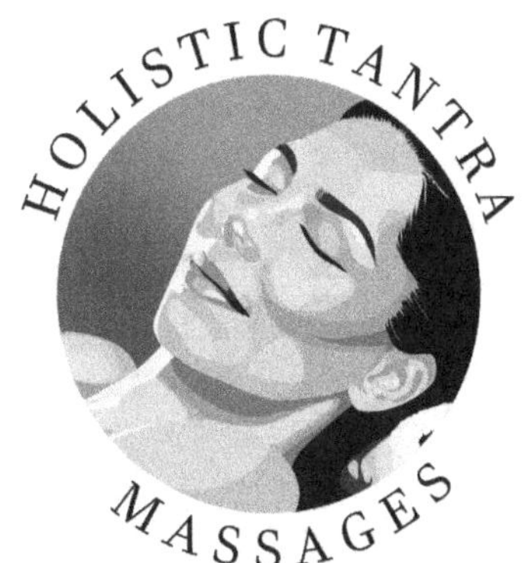

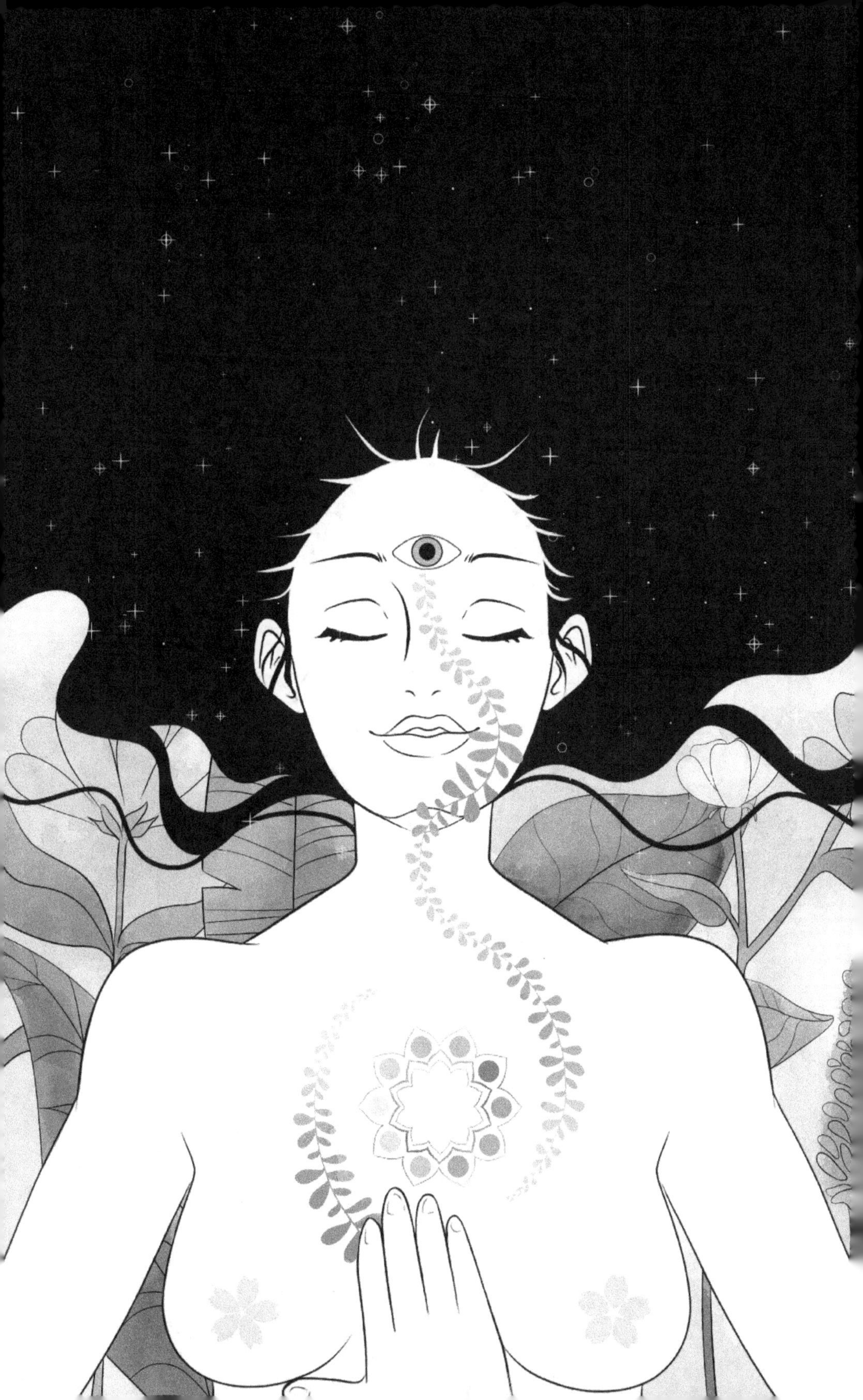

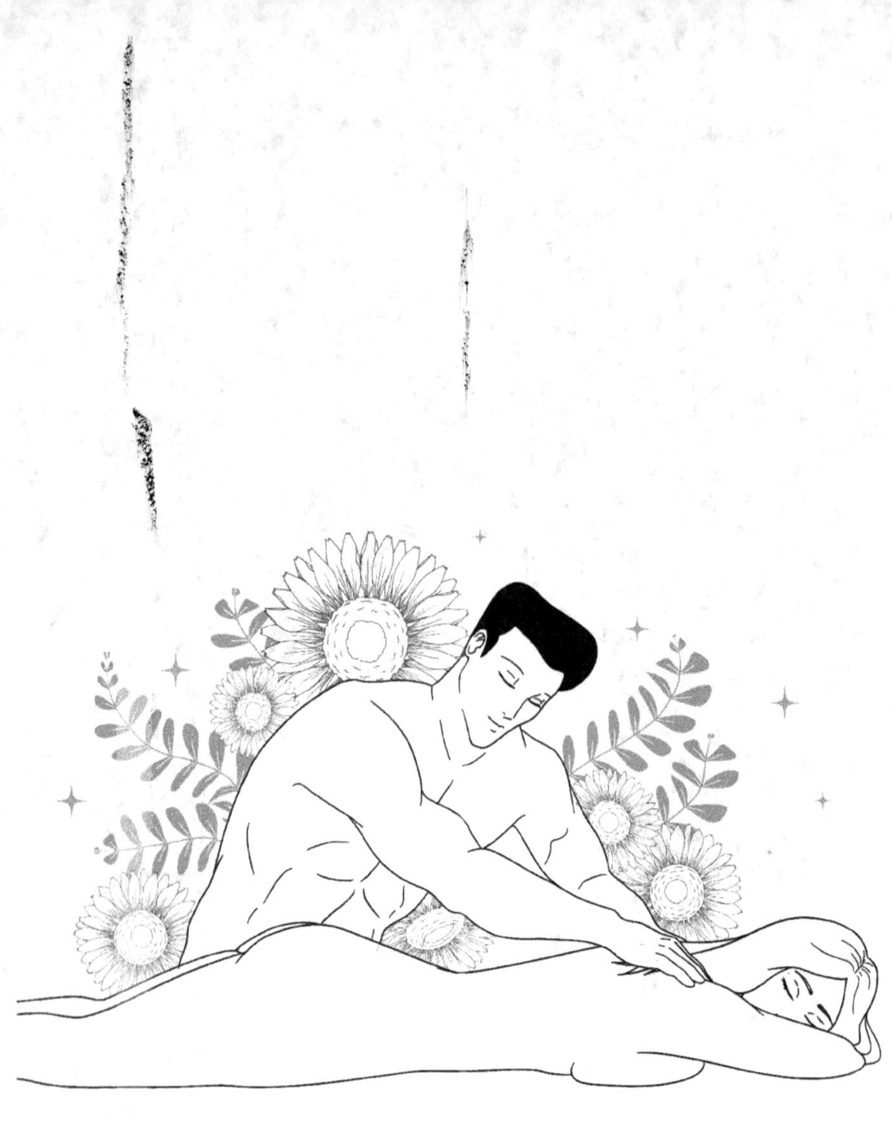

# Table of Contents

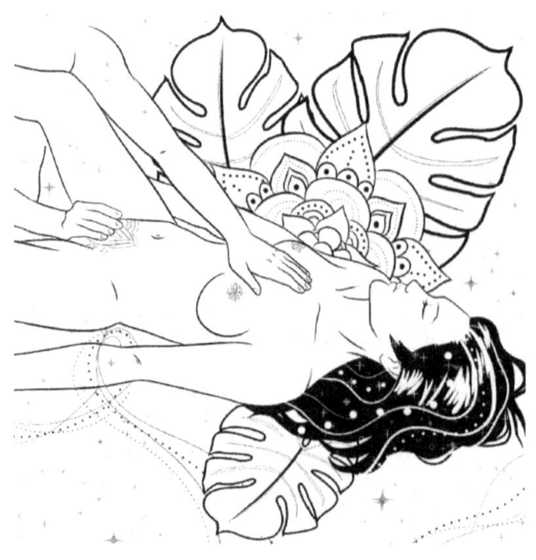

# Introduction

**M**odern society tends to limit the comprehension we have of our body and sexuality, often causing physical and emotional discomfort. **Tantric massages** invite us to re-discover the sacredness of the Being, promoting a deeper connection with our body and re-activating any potential sleeping or blocked energies.

You will learn more about the transformative power of tantra and Yoni massage through clear instructions not only aimed at promoting a deeper sense of pleasure but also the general emotional comfort for both who receive and practice it.

This detailed but simple and clear guideline will lead you through the best positions, movements, and emotional conditions to spread your power and energies. Complemented by more than 80 accurate images about all the postures and techniques, it facilitates the learning process even to the very beginners, while also providing new ideas to the more expert ones!

*You are about to read a step-by-step book intended to guide you through the correct practice of tantra and Yoni massage, designed especially for the well-being and needs of women.*

Rooted in the ancient Indian tradition, **women's tantra massage** focuses on the female body's energetic zones to release any physical and emotional block, promoting a state of balance, joy, vitality, and pleasure.

As an essential part of this practice, **Yoni massage** aims at stimulating the female genital area for a deeper sense of relaxation and wellness (in Sanskrit, the term "yoni" refers to the female entire reproductive system). For women, its benefits include greater body awareness, a reduced sense of stress, and an improvement in the reaching of the orgasm, to promote self-intimacy and with the partner too.

Here, you will find several topics intended to enrich your experience with Tantric Massages and to help you create a deeper connection with yourself, **awakening your kundalini energy**. We will talk about the best ways to balance your Chakras to boost your energies. You will learn how to create the perfect environment around you during your massages through the use of essential oils and gems. You will also find out more about breathing and meditation techniques for your physical and mental preparation.

You will explore Yoni's sacred anatomy, showing you how to improve your knowledge of your body and learn new massage techniques, as well as **how to stimulate and turn on the sexual tension through specific positions and movements, all this through a gradual, respectful but effective approach.** In addition to this, you will find a direct link at the end of the book so as for you to download the proper music track for your tantra and Yoni massage, for a way more special experience.

**Tantra Yoni massage offers you multiple incredible benefits, which do not concern the experience as a couple only, but the very individual person carrying it out too:**

1.      **Full attention on your partner:** by entirely focusing on your partner, you will get every day better at giving them love and pleasure, strengthening your bond.

2.      **A greater mutual understanding and connection:** it encourages deeper communication and a stronger emotional connection with your partner.

3.      **More satisfying sexual experiences:** By finding out which erogenous zones satisfy your partner the most, you will make your intimate life way more satisfactory for both of you.

4.      **A happier relationship:** making your partner happy with a good massage will bring much more joy and fulfillment to your relationship.

Every practice here described is the outcome of several years of study and experience in the field. You can also find our contacts at the end of the book; in case you need any further explanation or want to share your opinions and suggestions on the content.

*Enjoy your reading!*

# 1. A Guide to the Tantric Massage: What Is It and How Can It Make Your Life Better

Tantra massage, also commonly known as tantric massage, is not bound to a mere physical practice; indeed, it represents an improvement opportunity for your psychophysical well-being, allowing you to experience a true state of relaxation and listen to your body while getting lost in the moment. This sensorial experience is highly connected to the typical tantric vision of life, according to which every daily moment can be regarded as "tantric" if fully lived with the right awareness and involvement.

According to the ancient philosophical view, the material world represents the tangible manifestation of the intangible one, where the physical universe is the direct, visible expression of deeper and invisible forces or energies—acknowledging it and diving into the senatorial experience is the only way for a complete union with the invisible and for experiencing an inner state of peace and joy.

Nowadays, it is easier to feel distant from who and what surrounds us every day, losing our ability to smell fragrances, to feel in a state of trance in front of a humbling, beautiful sight, to feel lulled by the wind on our skin, or to enjoy the sun warming us and giving us light. This is why tantra teaches us to enjoy the "small joys of life," even though they represent what is most vital in our lives.

According to this, the reason why we end up relying on artificial sources of pleasure is that we are no longer able to live fully. **If only we could go back to that state of union with nature and people, we probably would no longer need to run after something else.** Tantra's main purpose is to lead us back to our origins, helping us to re-discover ourselves and be in control of our most hidden emotions, promoting both our mental and physical health while also positively influencing every other area of our life, to heal from our past wounds through pleasure.

Among the several Tantric practices, massage is particularly known for its ability to support the body in terms of senses stimulation and muscle relaxation. Also, this state of well-being is the direct result of the deep intimacy established between the massage giver and receiver. As a result, it generates an increased awareness of one's desires and emotions, being able to embrace the present without too many expectations or restrictions.

This is the heart of tantra: a path towards self-comprehension and a better understanding of what surrounds us, through connection and fellowship, to feel more grateful every day. Tantra represents the essence of everything around us, the vital energy we can perceive through our senses. However, we may tend to feel increasingly disturbed by what is around us rather than humbled by it. **Tantra shows us a way to find our center again, reconnecting with our energy and restoring our life balance.** It is a practice that constantly aims at challenging us to find our real purpose in life and bring us back to the original state of calm and gratitude.

Tantra mainly focuses on the vital energy, which is the so-called prana we get from what is outside of us, as well as on the sexual one, known as the kundalini energy, that is inside of us, and on the Shakti and Shiva main poles, respectively representing the female and male pole. Both of them are inside of us, whose goal is to find a union and a balance between them, being able to move, dance, and merge.

Through the tantric massage, we dig into a deep sensory experience meant to reconnect us to the beauty of our true nature, to take us to a new, higher level of consciousness.

*In the Tantric Massage, specific techniques are used to alternate a sense of intensity and softness, based on the breath rhythm and respecting the body's energy flows and chakras. What truly distinguishes this practice has to do with the inner attitude of the operator, supporting the receiver on their inner journey.*

In this type of massage, there is a specific role played by physical contact, since it takes on a profound cognitive value, going beyond mere manual technique. During the massage operator and receiver interaction, different levels of communication are established, starting with the physical dialogue, after the first meditative phase.

In all types of massages, there is always a sort of energy exchange, as it is in the tantric kind, where it is even more evident. During the practice, the touch itself acts on the body by generating several sensations and emotions not only involving the mind but also the innermost part of the being. Every movement is a loving caress that works as a gateway for a greater level of personal awareness, allowing the person undergoing the practice to rediscover the beauty that is in them, for a new inner world full of new sensations and perceptions. Every physical part conveys unique vibes that can be perceived as pleasant or annoying, according to each person's taste. Anyway, all these differences allow you to learn and understand more about yourself, exploring your body and every change you need to make for your personal improvement and well-being.

Despite the possible physical aversions or resistance, **the human being always has a deep need for love and affection, which is vital for psycho-physical well-being.** It concerns both men and women as an evident result of the message's importance when it comes to relationships and every human bond too. Ultimately, the body represents the main medium through which we are enabled to experience and understand the world, becoming a gateway to access our true Self. As a consequence, tantra massage is an extraordinary opportunity for immediate well-being and a long-lasting personal evolution.

During the massage, the particular hand movement skills lead to a deep awareness of each gesture and breath, facilitating self-understanding and the resolution of emotional blocks that have been withstanding your happiness and well-being in your everyday life. People receiving the massage usually notice a considerable change in their initial state of stiffness, starting to be able to listen to the sensations crossing their body again with a new, different perception. This reconnection can lead to unprecedented moments of joy and freedom, marking the beginning of a fresh path toward much more self-awareness.

During the massage, physical tensions are released and you can bump into eventual emotional blocks especially towards the end of the session, or even after. These experiences can be intense and do require adequate support by the person practicing it all, according to their role as spiritual guide for your body.

## The Benefits of the Tantric Touch: A Deep Connection

Tantra massage is not bound to a strict series of manual movements but tends to mainly focus on a different, important kind of touch which is not necessarily related to the hands, since it is the direct result of a predisposition of the heart, which must be properly developed. As mentioned above, **the tantric massage is known to be a particular contact, the so-called "tantric touch."** The latter is not defined by the specific movements performed during the massage (which are still important and must be well defined), but rather by the deep sensitivity that gets manifested during the contact itself. Its main goal is not just related to the mere act of performing it, but rather to the way it gets done. Therefore, the person carrying it out must be well prepared. But don't worry, **you don't have to be a guru or spiritual guide! Just be sure to be fully present in what you are doing, to be doing it with love and clarity.** At the end of the reading, I recommend you to carefully read this book twice or three times again, so as for you to finally be able to try and put what you've learned into practice, perhaps with your partner's support.

By the way, the receiver needs to be ready and willing to receive the massage. Also, remember that constant practice is vital to improve and deepen your understanding—it must be both sensual and meditative, designed to awaken the body's consciousness and connect with the deepest layers of the unconscious. It is essential that the practitioners of tantric massage not only master the techniques but also possess a deep inner sensitivity and connection with the very root of life.

**Tantric massage aims at releasing sexual energy, allowing it to freely flow in the body and experiencing a sense of lightness and sensitivity, which inevitably leads to a better knowledge of ourselves and our body.**

Although it is both technically and conceptually similar to the Californian massage, the tantric type is different in the importance it gives to the meditative aspect and the awakening of deep body consciousness. Nevertheless, if both types emphasize physical and emotional connection, the tantric one goes deeper and strives to lead to a state of total awareness.

Indeed, all the everyday concerns and stress we are likely to experience as humans are emotional tensions that are reflected in our body, stiffening our muscles, especially those belonging to the pelvis area for women, and compromising our normal approach to life. **Through Yoni tantric massage, tensions can be released, reducing stress and bringing great relief, relaxation, and mental peace**, which can be particularly useful for couples, as it helps to release accumulated tension and create an intimate atmosphere. Not only does taking time to do this improve the way you can give pleasure to your partner but also it is a great way to show them your respect and love.

Anyway, saying that it must be all done with love and tenderness for it to be truly considered an act of affection is an understatement, and this is the reason why it is best performed with someone you have a deep, authentic bond with since all your emotional commitment is required and fundamental.

Several benefits proceed from this practice and concern women, such as:

* Major body sensitivity to erogenous stimulations.
* Major self-confidence and body awareness, as well as that of your womanhood.
* A higher level of trust in the partner.
* Less frigidity, vaginal dryness, less sense of low libido, less frequent irregular period and cramps, as well as pain and vaginal irritation.
* Emotional openness to the partner, overcoming fears and limits.
* Bad memories are driven away to fully experience pleasure.
* Less post-menstrual tensions and irritability.
* Higher sexual pleasure.
* Freedom by repressed feelings, for a free-flowing of your energy.
* It helps you to be fully aware of your feelings. Moreover, the massage is also highly useful to the person carrying it out, since it allows an exclusive focus on the partner, improving the quality of the **sexual act and the level of harmony with your partner, enabling you to discover the erogenous zones that give more pleasure to the other,** to make the relationship more pleasant for both.

When I started studying the tantric kind of massage, one of the very first things my teacher taught me was that its true power does not only lie in caresses and touches; indeed, you might not even physically touch the other person, but still get the benefits by merely concentrating on visualizing the vital energy flowing through both of you.

As you feel your partner's body, just try to focus your attention on these forces and imagine having the power to move them and redirect them wherever you want to, according to the centers of energy. The main concept is related to the fact that **our hands must not be perceived as mere physical tools, but as sources of energy and heat,** as also demonstrated by the simple fact that, by pointing a thermograph at a human body, a cold and hot point can be spotted, with the latter particularly concentrated along the spine, which is the central axis of our being and the point where our energy centers reside, the seven chakras. **Therefore, the tantric touch is not just something physical, but also an act of focusing and energy shifting**

**that is the direct result of an attempt to rebalance and harmonize what is inside of us.** It is an experience in which the hand is also guided by the power of thought, which promotes a state of well-being to the body, but also to the energetic and emotional world. The tantric touch is more than a simple material action; indeed, it requires a much deeper intention, particular attention to breathing, and a special connection with the partner, also through meditation.

This is the reason why the tantric massage is often regarded as a ritual, for it goes beyond the material world and therefore cannot be taught simply through a book. However, we try to bring passionate and interested people in this field, like you, a bit closer. This reading represents just the beginning of a wider journey into the exploration of the tantric massage and tantra world more generally! We hope it can be a solid starting point for you and your personal and spiritual growth and that of your well-being.

The connection between the massager and the receiver is described as an interaction that goes beyond mere physical contact but also **involves an emotional and spiritual sphere.** This is the reason why the experience is not just good for the body, but also good for the soul. **Tantric massage is not just a series of physical movements, but something deeper involving the mind, body, and spirit.** It is an inner exploration process of ourselves and others.

After the massage, many people tend to feel a sense of rebirth and purification, along with joy and emotional freedom. This represents a form of deep release from the blocks and tensions that have been held within over time, to reach an authentic state of peace and self-exploration.

Osho, one of the greatest Indian spiritual mentors, has well explained the important concept of tantra in relation to tension release and full self-expression thanks to a state of harmony with the body and the sexual energies. Osho invites us to learn from animals, **especially cats, who live without any pressures and have a natural tendency to relax.** On the contrary, from the very childhood, all human beings are highly led to feel uncomfortable when dealing with sexuality, which is explained by Osho as a block causing a superficial kind of breathing in the body that withstands the free flowing of the sexual energy, leading to a lack of vitality and self-confidence and hindering the achievement of a high state of intelligence.

On the other hand, tantra proposes a total embrace of sexuality, by letting its energy flow freely without any kind of repression or conflict. It invites us to take care of our bodies and to recognize the importance of self-acceptance. Osho points out that the body should not be considered as a burden to bear, but rather as a **tool**

**for spiritual realization**, to love and accept and through which we can achieve a deeper inner harmony and, consequently, pave the way to a healthy way to love and take care of our dear ones.

Finally, he also points out that self-love is the foundation for every other kind of love. If we do not love and accept our body first, we will never be able to receive and accept love from others. Tantra practice consists of embracing our bodies completely every day by eliminating any form of judgment or self-condemnation, opening the door for a new kind of **freedom and spiritual realization.**

Even though it requires nakedness, it goes beyond the **simple act of taking off your clothes,** since it is simply a symbolic gesture representing the very first step towards self-acceptance and self-love, which is fundamental: only those who can accept and love themselves can fully live all the experiences and possibilities life wants to offer them.

When you first approach the practice, even if you are used to getting undressed without too much trouble, you can practice self-acceptance. Indeed, it is common for people, especially women, to feel uncomfortable while taking off their bra or while showing a certain part of their body they particularly feel insecure about, although it is necessary to remove everything completely to allow the massage to flow freely. Feeling confident with your body is the first step, and the massage begins when you decide to embrace the full experience, forgetting all of your insecurities.

For a full approach to your body, mind, and emotions, it is essential for you to carefully listen to yourself since it is you who is at the very center of the whole practice, and it is vital that your mind is fully present during the entire process and that you are truly aware of what is happening, for inner peace and silence to be guaranteed. Of course, all this requires a lot of attention, both in the environment you carry it all out and in the way you approach it, to make the other person feel welcomed and at ease during the massage. Indeed, your main purpose must be that of setting up a safe environment for your partner to freely explore their sensations and perceptions.

According to the tantric vision, the human body is sacred and none of its parts are forbidden to the Spirit to access, but must be taken into account in its fullness. However, modern society can be highly likely to limit our understanding, generating psychosomatic and existential discomfort. Hence, **tantric massage invites us to go back to the original state of sacredness of the Being,** making it possible for us to develop a deep connection with our Temple, which is our body, and inner being. It is important then to understand that there is no standard practice to follow or strict results to be obtained, as each experience is different and is linked to the present moment and the person involved.

Anyway, some ambiguities must be dispelled. Unlike the widespread belief, tantric massage does not only have a purely erotic purpose but is meant to represent an opportunity of spiritual value with a more evolutionary aim, **bringing way more benefits than what is thought and helping us to solve any psycho-affective and sexual discomfort.** Also, even though it was inspired by tantrism, it just shares the basic principles with it, applying them to the sphere of massage.

Tantrism is a spiritual and philosophical practice rooted in the ancient religious tradition of India and is characterized by its holistic and inclusive approach, which integrates spiritual, philosophical, and practical elements. In short, it aims at promoting the improvement of self-consciousness and the achievement of a state of "enlightenment" through a series of other practices involving meditation, yoga, rituals, mantras, and, in some cases, even multiple sexual aspects.

It is important to highlight, though, that Tantrism is not limited to the mere sexual sphere but includes a wide range of teachings aimed at inner transformation and spiritual awareness. However, it is to be understood that it must not be confused with the tantric practice itself, which is inserted in a holistic perspective and also sees sexuality as a means to reach ecstasy and spiritual elevation, as it is for the maithuna practice, which involves the spiritual union of two individuals. The term comes from Sanskrit and refers to a traditional practice of tantra related to a sacred and conscious kind of sexual union between two individuals whose main aim is to get to a state of ecstasy and spiritual elevation.

In the context of tantra, maithuna is considered a holy and transformative act, where sexual energy is used to achieve a deep state of awareness and spiritual connection between the two partners. Anyway, it is fundamental to stress how the practice is to be carried out within a spiritual and completely consensual context and must not be confused with common sexual practices or promiscuity, which is to be kept in mind due to several misleading and disrespectful massage offers presented as "tantric," **likely to affect women in particular, since more sensitive and closer to the topic.**

Tantra can also be often misinterpreted and be perceived as aimed at making the sexual act last longer, even though it is much deeper and more complex. According to the ancient Indian original term, *tantra* comes from Sanskrit and means "net" or "plot," but also "ritual," indicating a set of fields and spiritual teachings that have been developed over the centuries within Indian religions. These teachings have taken various shapes and have been influenced by different traditions, such as Hinduism, Buddhism, Jainism, etc., while also spreading to Tibet, China, and other parts of the Far East.

The concept itself is rooted in the Sanskrit word *tan*, which literally means "to lay the frame on the warp," in a broader sense in terms of expanding or dilating the Spirit, the unconditional consciousness, and the self, as opposed to the psychophysical ego. Therefore, the first step on your tantric path is the purification of the sensoriality, to free it from every kind of contamination from everyday life and develop a more refined perception ability. Through refined sensory experiences, such as colors, scents, sounds, and physical contact, we can live the present with a major intensity.

Even though tantric massage can become a meditative experience itself, opening your mind to the discovery of eternity from the present moment, it is essential to distinguish between authentic practices and common misunderstandings. Indeed, all of the practices can widely shift, from the more traditional to the most personal kinds, developed through direct and extended experiences.

Anyway, it is important to understand that tantra emphasizes the importance of feelings and emotions for authentic purposes and personal development, rather than for superficial or selfish goals. That being said, with the passing of time and the spread in the Western world, it is quite reasonable that the majority of tantra practices, teachings, and rituals have undergone a significant evolution, being adapted to Western people's mentality and habits. This has occurred quite naturally, as the way we perceive and integrate these disciplines is strongly influenced by our culture and perspectives.

In this context, for example, the tantric topic of pleasure and sex has often been emphasized, even though we have to keep in mind that **tantra's culture has spirituality at its center,** and the mental and spiritual energies are considered as tangible and vital aspects of the human being. This is the main reason why, despite accurate studies and insights, it is not always easy to fully grasp its true meaning and power. We will try to accurately synthesize some basic notions through a practical guide to integrate both the energetic and spiritual aspects of the massage.

However, the perception of these concepts will vary according to the sensitivity of the reader. If some might grasp both the practical-concrete and spiritual aspects, others might tend to prefer just the first ones. Nevertheless, we have to portray the tantric massage for what it is as a whole, without neglecting the more abstract aspect, but while also taking our pragmatic and Western approach into account, focusing then **on the "technical" aspect of one of the tantric disciplines, which is to say, tantra and yoni massage** (as essentials).

It is also important to remark that tantra, and the tantric massage in particular, cannot be entirely learned from a book, but it is something to transmit directly, even though the books available are quite good at providing detailed information.

Personally, as a holistic practitioner, I have studied, deepened, and practiced massage in different parts of the world, getting to observe people's multiple motivations and expectations to approach it. If some people are seeking a kind of transgression, others simply wish to experience something new and inspiring, while others are fully aware of the kind of experience they are going to live and want to dig into it with all of their mind and spirit, deciding to experience it together as a couple to learn all of the techniques and rituals to apply to their intimacy. This way, the massage not only becomes a moment of shared pleasure, but also an opportunity to explore, and enrich the relationship itself. This is what I will be trying to do through this guide providing you with all that you need to repeat and live what you will learn here!

# Feel It Again with Your Kundalini Primal Energy

Through a tantric massage, we aim at stimulating all of our senses, among which the most developed one nowadays is sight. The main purpose is to rebalance our energy centers by mainly activating that of the heart, which can be achieved either through a gentle and loving approach or **through the more direct awakening of the sexual energy, kundalini.** Kundalini is a traditional Hindu concept, present in both yoga and tantra, which must be awakened through massage as well as the energy that is within us. It is a primordial kind of energy that, according to the yogic and tantric traditions, is located at the base of the spine, and its awakening can lead to a way greater spiritual awareness, emotional balance, and psycho-physical well-being.

This vital energy can be a source of intense and pleasant sensations when stimulated and is often represented as a sleeping snake. According to Hindu belief, it can be awakened and raised along the spine, where there is a channel called *Sushumna*, through various spiritual and meditative practices such as yoga, meditation, and tantra massage. When the Kundalini is awakened, it begins to flow through the body like a rushing river, following the movement as a snake towards the upper part of the body, ready to clean up and purify all the chakras, to open them and unlock them. However, in some cases, it could bump into some emotional blocks along the path, where the full attention and presence of the massage giver are required, fully ready to grapple with possible conflicting, emotional reactions such as sudden laughter, anger, or sadness, as these can be manifestations of the blocked energy.

Indeed, when performing a tantric massage, whether to your partner, to a friend, or a client, **the most important thing is to be fully present in the moment, to establish a deep spiritual and energetic connection,** while also taking into account that not all of the people you will interact with will be as sensitive as the same. When the kundalini awakens and rises along the energy channel, you are leading the other person to a state of enlightenment and connection with the divine and spiritual realization, but if it is not properly managed, can cause physical, emotional, and mental problems.

The concept of kundalini is also present in many other spiritual traditions, although with slightly different names and concepts. For example, in the Chinese tradition, it is similar to the concept of Qi, while in Tibetan Buddhism it is associated with that of *tummo* (inner heat). **Sexual energy is considered one of the most powerful forms of physical energy humans can experience**, capable of transforming our existence and spreading into all the other dimensions of the being.

In the ancient Eastern traditions, there are specific massage techniques properly thought for the genitals, known as **lingam massage for men and Yoni massage for women.** They require complex and articulated manual skills, which is very different from the view that we have of it as Western countries. In general, the tantric massage provides a powerful sensory experience for meditative purposes, well-being, and personal growth, being an experience accessible to all, which can be both part of a path of personal development or simply a moment of relaxation and well-being. **It can also offer benefits for specific sexual problems, such as anorgasmia or arousal difficulty,** becoming integrative support for specific therapies followed by specialists.

# About the author

Behind "Holistictantramassages" lies Den Damant, a holistic practitioner from Milan with a deep passion for well-being, which he cultivates through holistic and tantric practices. For the past four years, Den has dedicated himself to the practice of massage and beyond, continuously refining his techniques and expanding his knowledge through studies and updates on complementary disciplines.

A year ago, Den decided to share his experience through books and social media, founding the page "@holistictantramassages" and publishing his first book, *Tantra Yoni Massage: The Dance of Ecstasy*, still under the pseudonym Holistictantramassages. This work offers a practical and profound guide for those who wish to discover the sacred power of tantric massage for women. His goal is to make this page and his books a point of reference for anyone wanting to explore the holistic and tantric world.

Through this space, Den shares useful advice and inspiration for relaxing the mind and body, promoting an authentic and conscious approach to well-being and personal growth. This page is not just a stopping point; it is a true reference point for anyone wishing to immerse themselves in a journey of personal growth and holistic well-being. With rich and valuable content, Den offers suggestions, techniques, and inspiration for relaxing both body and mind, making an holistic approach to well-being accessible to all—one that goes beyond the surface and can transform lives once discovered.

Whether you are a novice to tantra or a long-time explorer of the holistic world, this book has something to offer you. Den's journey is not just a personal quest but an invitation for everyone to pause, breathe, and rediscover their potential through greater self-awareness of their body and soul.

If you want to go beyond the simple concept of well-being and feel that there is something deeper to explore, then you are in the right place. Let yourself be inspired by Den and his journey, and begin your path toward a new dimension of well-being, where every moment becomes an opportunity to grow, heal, and connect with the most authentic essence of yourself.

# 2. Align Your Seven Chakras: The Power of the Massage Through Kundalini and Prana

Tantra massage works primarily through two forces: prana, the vital energy that permeates everything around us, and kundalini, which, as we have mentioned before, is a kind of relict energy that comes from creation and is found within us, flowing through the chakras. The person carrying out the massage must be full of prana energy to fully connect and share it with the other person. In fact, prana is a key word in the philosophy of yoga and the ancient Indian tradition, coming from Sanskrit and roughly translatable as a "vital breath," or a "universal life force." Through contact, stimulation, and full attention, the massager guides the energy through the chakras, which get awakened and rebalanced, allowing the power to flow freely and rekindle the inner flame.

## Prana: The Vital Essence That Permeates the Universe

When talking about prana, we refer to something more than simple energy but rather to a manifestation of the divine itself. Indeed, it gives life to the universe and represents the breath that animates every form of existence, as well as the air we breathe.

At the heart of tantra massage, prana becomes a love dance and a celebration of life itself, one of the main reasons why it is commonly considered as **the life energy or force that permeates the entire universe and animates every form of life.**

According to yoga, it is considered the basis of everything because it circulates through subtle channels called nadi, part of the subtle energy body known as the "energy layer," and can be influenced and balanced through yoga practices such as breathing, physical postures, meditation, and concentration. The concept is also linked to several other spiritual and philosophical traditions, such as Ayurveda (the system of traditional Indian medicine), Tibetan Buddhism, and the ancient Vedic philosophy, where prana is considered a key element for physical, mental, and spiritual health.

**Tantra not only sees prana as a vital force, but also as a powerful cognitive and energetic tool,** able to deeply influence our bodily, mental, and spiritual experience. This essential aspect of the practice cannot be overlooked, and even though some concepts may seem abstract to many, it is important to understand that, since this book focuses on tantra and Yoni massage, it is my duty to bring to light its true spiritual meaning. It is not about the simple act of performing a massage, but it is more about **honoring and reckoning what the soul is by an exploration of its emotional and energetic influences on the body, considered as the sacred temple of the massage receiver.**

# Kundalini: How to Awaken Your Sleeping Sexual Energy

During the tantric massage, the seven chakras are stimulated. The practice starts with the heart chakra, as its opening facilitates the flow of energy through the main channel, known as Sushumna nadi. This is crucial to allow the energy to rise from the base of the spine to the top of the head.

Tantric techniques may include gentle pressures, circular movements, and light touches along the points of the chakras, helping to release the energy blocks and promote the free-flowing of it all. After the heart chakra, the focus shifts to the vertebral area, where the stimulations are aimed at letting kundalini energy circulate along the entire spine, from the coccyx to the crown of the head.

This can lead to a gradual awakening of kundalini that is manifested through sensations of warmth, vibrations, and a sense of expansion, undergoing a profound inner transformation, improving self-awareness, a sense of creativity, and vitality.

Another important aspect of the tantric massage is the ability of the vital energy to transform into a sexual one. This does not necessarily include sexual activity, but a kind of integration of it as part of our overall life energy.

In the following chapters, we will dig into the exploration of the best way to perform a massage, **discovering the directions of movements, the intensity of the pressures, and the specific techniques to stimulate the chakras and release the energy blocks, for each movement and touch will have a determinant role in the awakening of the sleeping energy!**

Each chapter will be full of detailed and practical instructions, which will guide you on a step-by-step journey towards the rediscovery of your kundalini. Illustrations and descriptions will be provided for each technique, enabling you to immediately put into practice all that you have learned.

This knowledge will help you develop a complete and conscious practice, capable of profoundly transforming your inner energy and overall well-being!

## The Seven Chakras: The Primal Energy Vortexes in the Human Body

As anticipated before, the chakras are energy vortices located in so-called "subtle bodies," which is to say, energy layers surrounding us with specific characteristics and functions. They fluctuate, absorb energies from the outside to the inside, and expel them back again, allowing us to live in harmony with every aspect of our existence, and if something disturbs this balance, the massage contributes to the return to the initial state of balance and well-being, overcoming any obstacle with grace and calmness.

According to the tantric practice, the seven energy points represent vital energy vortices in the human body meant to regulate organic, mental, and emotional functions. According to the oriental philosophies that explore the concept of life flow that runs through our being, all this is based on these centers, since it is also already well-known that energy is fundamental for us to perform all of our daily activities, such as walking or eating. Not only does this energy get transformed into creative power, but also in a surprising sexual one!

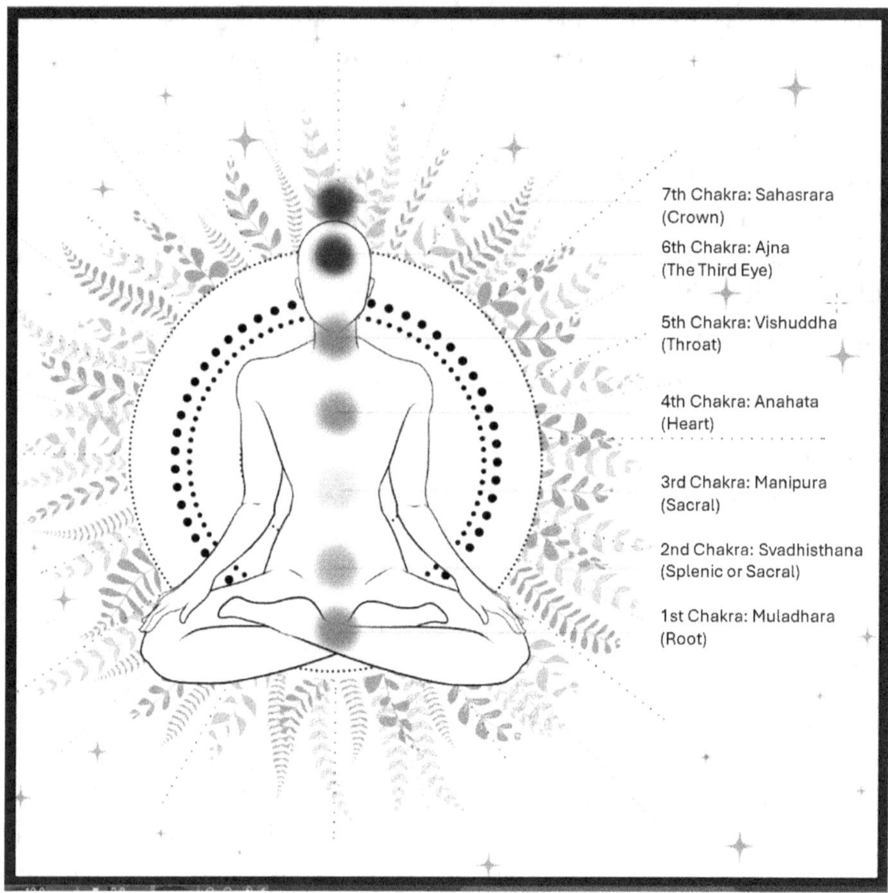


## First Muladhara Chakra — Root

**The first chakra (trust)** is located at the base of our spine, its predominant color is red and **the associated element is earth.** Associated with it are the adrenal glands, which are located above the kidneys, as well as the root, overseeing the production of stress hormones. The related organ of sense is the nose, linked to our smell and connected to the more primitive functions of the brain. This chakra is energetically linked to our legs, feet, bones, rectum, fatty intestine, immune system, and teeth as far as the physical body is concerned.

As for its connection with the energy and mental body, it represents the vitality of the body, constituting the foundation of mental and emotional health, as well as the psychological one. Somehow, it also concerns the process of childbirth, the perpetuation of the species, family connections, ties, and traditions, which influence a person's identity and sense of belonging and their ability to take care of themselves and face the challenges of life, as well as the ability to support their reasons. The primary function of the first chakra is rooting, which is the connection of the physical body to planet Earth. When it is unbalanced, its negative results are instability, physical, emotional, and working weakness, insecurity, lack of confidence and determination, and difficulty in building important things in life on solid foundations, as well as other symptoms such as aggression, impulsivity, chronic pain in the lower back, sciatica, varicose veins, hemorrhoids, intestinal disorders, depression, and immune system problems.

## Second Svadhisthana Chakra—Splenic or Sacral

The second chakra is located in the lower region of our abdomen, below the navel, and its color is orange, whilst the associated element is water, and the gonads are the glands involved. When it comes to its connection to the physical body, it involves the abdomen, genitals, kidneys, bladder, large intestine, pelvis, and lumbar vertebrae, whilst on the emotional and mental level it influences our interactions with others, our sexual desire, level of creativity and emotions, and these are some of the reasons why its primary function is related to interpersonal relationships, sexual pleasure, and emotional expression. Its dysfunction can inevitably cause relational problems, difficulties in social interaction, addiction, hot flashes, post-menstrual syndrome, fibroids, prostate disorders, circulatory problems, lower back pain, urinary disorders, and a general feeling of fatigue.

## Third Manipura Chakra—Sacral

The third chakra, located in the solar plexus area, between the navel and the sternum, is represented with a bright yellow color and is associated with the element of fire. The glands involved include the pancreas and adrenal glands, its energetic connection with the physical body concerns the stomach, gallbladder, liver, spleen, and the part of the spine behind the solar plexus and its main function has to do with the regulation of the metabolism and human personality and ego, determining our self-expression. It tackles fear, self-confidence, and how we confidently deal with complex situations. It aims at fully expressing personal power and if it does not properly work in us, we can face difficulties in making decisions, overcoming challenges, communicating our needs to others, feeling misunderstood with outbursts of anger, and also leading to digestive problems, metabolic disorders, diabetes, constipation, parasitic infestations, nervousness, and weakened memory.

## Fourth Anahata Chakra — Heart

The fourth chakra is located at the center of the chest and is linked to the colors green and pink. Its element is the air, while the involved gland is the thymus. Its energetic connection with the physical body concerns the heart, the circulatory system, ribs, breast, lungs, shoulders, arms, hands, and diaphragm, whilst on the emotional and mental level it is responsible for the way our emotions are controlled, as well as for the ability to let go and surrender what we cannot control and freedom from emotional pain through the healing energy of forgiveness. The fourth chakra is the center of compassion and love, acting as a bridge between body and mind, earth and heaven. Its dysfunctions can manifest with cardiac arrhythmias, heart attacks, asthma, allergies, pain in the shoulders and upper back, breast and lung cancer, and bronchopneumonia.

## Fifth Vishuddha Chakra — Throat

The fifth chakra is located in the throat region and is represented by a clear blue color. It is characterized by the element of air and the gland involved is the thyroid. Its energetic connection with the physical body concerns the throat, thyroid, trachea, esophagus, parathyroid, hypothalamus, cervical vertebrae, mouth, jaws, and teeth, and on an emotional and mental level, it promotes the ability to follow your dreams, make decisions, and maintain the determination to achieve them. It is the center of connection with the divine, of faith and surrender, and it controls, creates, transmits, and receives communication through sounds and vibrations, facilitating self-expression and creativity. The dysfunctions of the fifth chakra can manifest with irritations and inflammations of the throat, laryngitis, thyroid problems, mouth ulcers, gum disorders, swelling of the glands, and problems with the temporomandibular joint, as well as scoliosis.

## Sixth Ajna Chakra — The Third Eye

It is located on the forehead and is characterized by an indigo color. It is connected to the light element and the gland involved is the pineal one. Its energetic connection with the body concerns the brain, the nervous system, the pineal gland, eyes, ears, and nose, and on the emotional and mental level, it is the center of intuition and knowledge, the source of introspection and wisdom, which allows us to see with the eyes of our soul and have full access to clairvoyance and intuition. The dysfunctions associated with this chakra include blindness, problems with the eye orbit, headaches, tension in the eyes, blurred vision, disorders of the spine, learning difficulties, tumors, hemorrhages, and cerebral strokes.

## Seventh Sahasrara Chakra—Crown

The last chakra is located on top of the head and its colors are purple and white. The element that represents it is thought, while the gland involved is the pituitary. As for the energetic connection with our body, this chakra is the gateway to the vital force coming from the divine and involves both the physical and mental bodies, both spiritual and energetic. Emotionally and mentally speaking, it stores the energy generated by prayer and meditation and is the energetic center of spiritual introspection and awareness. It is the source of cosmic consciousness and enlightenment, and its dysfunctions can manifest through energetic disorders, mystical crises, chronic fatigue, and extreme sensitivity to light, noise, and other environmental factors.

Chinese philosophy states that there is a flow of vital energy in the body's meridians, which is similar to the circulatory system that ensures organic well-being. Possible blocks in this flow can cause disorders and diseases that can be interpreted as signs of imbalance. The energy points along these meridians are similar to stations and can be stimulated to regulate the body's energy. These affect the functioning of the whole body, requiring a constant check to ensure the general well-being.

In traditional Chinese medicine, the concept of "energy meridians" can be linked to the chakra system of the ancient Indian tradition. Both systems focus on the vital energy that flows through the body and affects the physical, emotional, and mental realm, with the chakras being the only energy points extending along the spine and corresponding to different parts of the body, along with the meridians as channels through which this energy flows. Anyway, it is important to underline that the chakras are not the only energy centers in our bodies since many others are also present. However, we will mainly focus on these seven, as they are the most useful ones in the context of tantric massage.

Indeed, activating the chakras and experiencing an energy flow is beneficial to the massage. This way, the person carrying it out will be able to offer a more effective treatment, while the receiver will perceive their body more completely. Let's see a first, simple technique to activate them:

Sit down and cross your legs, put your hands on your knees or in another comfortable position, and focus on the first chakra, breathing and making ten cycles of inspiration and exhalation.

Breathing through a chakra means focusing on the area in which it is located, imagining to inhale and exhale from that point. You can breathe through your nose in both phases or inhale from the nose and exhale from the mouth, and after a few breaths, shift your attention to the second chakra, located just below the navel, and repeat the breathing cycle. Keep going until the seventh one, and once you have completed the cycles, keep focusing on your breath. Lie down and relax, taking some time to feel the effects of the exercise.

# 3. Prepare the Perfect Atmosphere Through the Four Elements and the Five Senses

## *How to Prepare What Is Outside and Inside of Us*

Before performing a tantric massage, it is essential to create a sacred space through careful preparation of both the external and internal environment. **The preparation of the external environment** includes the dedicated area to the massage and the altar (if there is no altar, take into account the zone around the point where the massage will be performed), also considering the four elements and the five senses. **The preparation of the internal space** has to do with an emotional kind of preparation, for both the massage giver and receiver, thanks to the breathing technique related to the chakras.

**The preparation of the external environment** includes everything that is outside of us, around us, such as walls, curtains, the futon, objects present in the room, lights (soft and indirect), a warm and comfortable temperature, etc. It is always advisable to have objects representing the four elements in the place where the massage will take place. Use inspiring, calming objects for your temple, along with symbols of the four elements:

- **Earth:** A stone.
- **Fire:** A lit white candle, preferably on a white plate.
- **Air:** A feather or a natural incense.
- **Water:** A water bowl with petals on the inside.

You can also add a statue or an image representing a Hindu deity or a particular figure you feel deeply connected to.

As for the five senses:

- **Sight:** Make sure the space is visually pleasant, with a good and indirect light system. The person receiving the massage may appreciate a nice decoration or a comfortable dressing gown!
- **Hearing:** It is important to have a relaxing, low-volume kind of background music.
- **Smell:** Incense, fresh flowers, and essential oils are important components. Avoid chemical fragrances and opt for natural ones, such as patchouli.
- **Taste:** Offer fruit, dried fruits, natural teas, water, and chocolate during breaks.
- **Touch:** Touch is key! Make sure your hands are soft and smooth, take care of your nails, and moisturize your hands with a cream. During the massage, be aware and gentle; use a natural oil, like almond or coconut oil, as it will immediately come into contact with the receivers' intimate areas; avoid chemical oils and go for natural ones, that are way more gentle and beneficial for the skin. You can also use a scarf, a feather, or particular stones to slide over the receiver's body by massaging it, creating immense pleasure.
- **Purification:** The person receiving the massage should take a shower (not too hot), avoiding deodorants and chemical fragrances.

When you welcome the woman, be gentle and speak as little as possible: start by calmly closing your eyes and connecting with your inner divinity and that of the other. Only after this initial inner contact, the massage can begin.

It is advisable to perform the massage on a futon, easily available on the market in various dimensions, avoiding those that are too thin as they may not be soft enough. **The space where the massage is to be performed must be extremely comfortable, with a proper surface to accommodate both the receiver and the giver's bodies, who will move around it.** A futon roughly 6 feet long (180 cm) and 5.2 feet wide (160 cm) would be simply perfect, but even one with slightly smaller sizes can fit. However, it is not advisable to use a too narrow one, such as one only 3 feet wide (90 cm), and it is also advisable to use a heating resistance to be placed under the futon, especially during the coldest seasons, to promote relaxation, as well as a sarong or some towels to be placed under it, to further improve comfort and hygiene during massage.

**Preparing your inner environment** means becoming fully aware of your emotional and mental state before starting the massage, which can be facilitated by practicing conscious breathing exercises and meditation, to develop a deep connection with yourself and others. It is also important to spend some time contemplating your body, spirit, and intentions to bring it all into the massage, focusing on leaving all the worries and tensions out.

Whether it is in a house, in a natural environment or any other place, it is essential to create a sacred space free from distractions and worries. This includes clearing your mind of negative thoughts, entirely focusing on the massage. Finally, this is all about a process of self-reflection and emotional purification, allowing both the massage giver and the receiver to fully get lost in the experience, creating a place of connection and mutual healing.

# The Perfect Essential Oils for Each Chakra

As said before, essential oils can be used to scent our environment during the massage, adding them to a dehumidifier or other electrical device that humidifies the air, to allow the aromas to spread throughout the room. It is also possible to add them to the same oil used for the massage itself, as essential oils have healing qualities, as well as aromatics that can bring specific benefits depending on the type. Below, is a list of essential oils recommended by the holistic discipline to promote the well-being of each chakra.

## To Support the First Chakra

To support the development of the first chakra, here are some essential oils that perfectly fit with this energetic center:

- **Vetyver:** Extracted from the roots, it represents nourishment, regeneration, and stability, helping to cope with emotional trauma and providing calm during high moments of tension and anxiety. It promotes emotional balance, the nervous system, the hormonal well-being, and also lowers blood pressure.
- **Nardo:** This essential oil promotes peace, serenity, and forgiveness, helping us to free ourselves from past traumas and emotional attachments. It also aligns our energies with what really matters, bringing stability to thoughts and feelings and supporting the circulatory system, hormonal balance, and iron absorption, which is beneficial during menopause, migraines, and insomnia.

- **Olibanum (incense):** Known for its calming properties, it connects our body to earth while also facilitating a connection with the divine light. It helps to drive earthly negativity away, promoting a sense of love and protection, and sorting conflicts out, while also relieving possible tensions, reducing mental fatigue, and strengthening the immune system. It is also valuable for arthritis and joint stiffness.
- **Myrrh:** It calms and soothes intense emotions, acting as a balm for both physical and emotional wounds, helping to let go of pain and suffering, especially during moments of anxiety and pressure. Myrrh also helps to restore the bond with Mother Earth, nourishing the relationship between mother and daughter.
- **Sandalwood:** Thanks to its balancing properties, it provides stability during moments of crisis or significant changes.

## To Support the Second Chakra

- **Sweet Orange:** It stimulates creativity, boosting our mood, and helping us during transition periods. It promotes contact with our inner child, promoting playfulness, lightheartedness, and joy, whilst also being beneficial for our digestion, immune system, and emotional balance of the skin.
- **Mandarin:** Particularly useful for improving our sense of abundance, especially when feeling down or hopeless. It promotes our sense of sharing and helps us to always find a solution with a positive effect on our digestion, immune system, and emotional balance.
- **Rose:** Being good for the heart chakra, the rose is the seed of life and the symbol of love. It is an aphrodisiac; a soothing and a good hormonal balancer. It regulates the metabolism of our heart and our dietary and sexual needs, reducing stress and helping to release excessive thoughts, while also being highly beneficial for our emotional balance and skin.
- **Jasmine:** Also useful for the heart chakra, jasmine is the oil of purity. It fights taboos and helps those who have received a too strict and puritanical education.
- **Ylang Ylang:** Suitable for the heart chakra too, it reduces our stress and boosts our mood, being an antidote to anger and aggression. It helps to dissolve limiting beliefs and problems resulting from a rigid education, bringing serenity and promoting relaxation.

## To Support the Third Chakra

- **Ginger:** It stimulates the will, promoting more courage and strength to act. It helps us focus on our goals and overcome the victimization feeling, promoting self-expression and self-confidence.
- **Grapefruit:** It withstands egocentrism and addiction by promoting self-esteem and self-acceptance, bringing light, and cleaning every blocked energy. It is useful for those who suffer from nervous hunger, and it promotes self-love and respect. It has a positive effect on the cardiovascular system.
- **Rosemary:** It promotes authority and fights apathy and inertia. It helps us to focus on our goals, and it is beneficial for our nervous and respiratory systems.
- **Bergamot:** It helps those who have low self-esteem to accept themselves and release repressed emotions, overcoming anxiety, sadness, and depression. It eliminates negative judgments and promotes emotional balance, with a positive effect on the digestive system and skin.
- **Copaiba:** It is useful against guilt, shame, or the sense of inadequacy, since it promotes self-forgiveness and acceptance, freeing us from negative emotions and helping us to live with a purpose while growing and improving. It has a beneficial effect on the cardiovascular, respiratory, nervous, muscular, bone, emotional, and skin systems.

## To Support the Fourth Chakra

- **Melissa:** This essential oil is renowned for its ability to reconnect with our divine essence, as it promotes emotional and mental balance, protecting us from negative external energy and freeing us from emotional addictions. It is known to convey enthusiasm and joy while acting positively on emotional balance and skin health.
- **Neroli:** It is an essential oil aimed at promoting a deep heart and soul connection, especially during moments of intimacy. It brings more harmony to the heart and calmness into a relationship, encouraging self-love and the perception of inner and outer beauty. It fights emotional pain and disorders such as panic, suffering, and depression while contributing to the well-being of the digestive system and skin.
- **Lavender:** It is known for its balancing power and is an important way to deal with anxiety, fear, sadness, and depression. It promotes kindness, understanding, and forgiveness, bringing calm, peace, and serenity, helping to overcome shyness, and contributing to the well-being of the nervous and cardiovascular system and the maintenance of emotional balance.

- **Geranium:** It heals our hearts and emotions, promoting love and forgiveness. It expresses the emotional pain we repress, opening our hearts to the possibility of loving again, contributing to the rebalancing of the nervous system, facing anxiety, fear, and depression, and also intensifying our perception, to shift our attention from what is rational to the heart, while positively acting on emotional balance and skin health.

## To Support the Fifth Chakra

- **Blue chamomile:** It promotes communication and spiritual awareness, stimulating intuitive abilities and helping to reveal the truth. It is an ally to cope with stress and communication difficulties.
- **Juniper berries:** They purify the physical and energetic body, protecting us from external influences and promoting mental clarity. It helps to get rid of negative thoughts and limiting beliefs, bringing peace and tranquility.
- **Cypress:** A symbol of stability and security, it promotes a balanced kind of self-expression and the ability to sort problems out. It helps to retain words and communicate harmoniously, while also being beneficial for the cardiovascular and musculoskeletal systems.
- **Eucalyptus:** It harmonizes the fifth chakra and promotes communication and self-expression, calming all sorts of agitation, giving faith, confidence, and inner strength, promoting mental clarity and the free movement of breath. It is also a support for the respiratory system and skin.

## To Support the Sixth Chakra

- **Scleraian Sage:** This essential oil is the perfect ally for those seeking mental clarity and vision since it helps to overcome a narrow-minded vision, opening the mind to new ideas and perspectives. It promotes psychological balance, providing mental clarity and emotional support during times of uncertainty.
- **Lemon:** It is a powerful tool for mental awakening since it frees the mind from mental blocks and stimulates consciousness and awareness. It is a symbol of confidence, optimism, and joy, perfect for those who desire a new beginning and greater mental clarity!
- **Lavender:** Known for its calming properties, the essential oil of lavender is also a powerful ally for inner freedom. It works on senses of insecurity and improved self-expression, helping to free ourselves from the fear of rejection. It promotes concentration and gratitude, for a major sense of inner peace and emotional well-being.

- **Marjoram:** It is particularly useful to withstand mental weariness and insomnia as it dissipates fear and confusion, offering mental clarity and inner calm. It frees the mind from limiting mental patterns and vicious circles, promoting relaxation and deep rest.

## To Support the Seventh Chakra

- **Incense:** Renowned for its properties of spiritual elevation and connection with the divine.
- **Benzoin:** It promotes contemplation and inner reflection, offering a sense of peace and serenity.
- **Jasmine:** It promotes an open mind and heart, facilitating access to deep meditative states.
- **Myrrh:** Known for its purifying and spiritual protection properties, it promotes awareness and mental clarity.
- **Sandalwood:** It improves inner calmness and mental peace, facilitating the connection with our spirituality.
- **Spruce:** It brings a sense of stability, helping to connect with the earthly and heavenly energy.
- **Lavender:** With its calming properties, it promotes inner peace, and relaxation during meditation.
- **Rose:** As a symbol of universal love and compassion, it promotes emotional healing, and the opening of the heart.
- **Basil:** It stimulates the mind and body, promoting concentration, and awareness during spiritual practice.
- **Rosemary:** Known for its properties of mental clarity and purification, it helps to get rid of negative thoughts, and energy blocks.
- **Angelica:** It promotes spiritual protection and openness to higher dimensions of awareness.
- **Star anise:** With its relaxing properties, it helps to release tensions and anxieties, facilitating the connection with the divine.
- **Blue chamomile:** It promotes tranquility and serenity, fostering a state of deep relaxation during meditation.
- **Gerani:** With its sweet and floral aroma, it helps to elevate the spirit, and cultivate feelings of gratitude and joy.

In order to use these essential oils and harmonize the crown chakra, you can spread the recommended oils during meditation or smell them directly from the bottle, to stimulate the senses. You can also pour a drop of it on your hands before starting meditation or relaxation exercises, allowing their healing properties to permeate your being and your partner.

# How to Use the Oils During a Massage and More

According to the holistic discipline, essential oils are a valuable resource for balancing our chakras and promoting energy harmony. Let's see together how to properly use them, even beyond the mere tantric practice!

Essential oils can be mixed with a carrier oil, such as coconut or sweet almond, to dilute them before their application on the skin, during the massage, which allows the aromas to be spread while benefiting from the therapeutic and healing properties of the oils. However, it is important to follow the recommended dilution indications and be careful of any possible allergy or skin sensitivity. After this, gently put them on the chakras' corresponding zones, and before applying them, take a moment to reflect and clarify the treatment intention. Remember to keep a clear focus on the chakra's purpose you are dealing with, since the use of essential oils can be enhanced if combined with proper mental focus during the session.

The best time to apply them is in the evening, especially before going to sleep, which allows them to act effectively on our unconscious side, promoting deep relaxation and the restoration of energy balance. Remember that the Chakras are closely related to the organs and emotional states, and although essential oils can provide temporary relief, it is also essential to address the underlying causes of discomfort for lasting benefits.

For each chakra, choose the appropriate oils and mix them with a carrier one, like almond oil. A diluted mixture allows deeper penetration and more effective action, and if you want to treat a single chakra more deeply, try using an essence diffuser. Add a few drops of the essential oil you want to use and stay focused before spreading the aromatherapy energy into the environment. Prepare your mixes in advance and store them in ready-to-use containers, to always have them ready for your treatments and at hand.

Deepen your wellness experience by integrating these techniques with meditation, yoga, and other holistic exercises. It is essential to pay particular attention to the fact that the oils must not come into contact with the mucous membranes, as they can cause irritation or unpleasant sensations. **When massaging the inner parts during a Yoni massage, it is always advisable to use natural oils without essential ones, such as sweet almond or coconut oil, since they are gentle on the skin and less likely to cause unwanted reactions. This approach ensures a safe and pleasant experience for the receiver of the massage.**

# The Most Suitable Gems for Each Chakra

As anticipated, it is possible to use stones during the massage. These can be placed in our "little temple" prepared for the massage, but also in contact with our body, worn as pendants, or passed along the body. Below, we propose a list of stones recommended by the holistic discipline to promote the well-being of each chakra.

## To Support the First Chakra

- **Obsidian:** Known for its physical rooting properties, it is particularly suitable for dealing with ailments such as arthritis and joint pain. This gem teaches us to flow and expand ourselves, freeing us from self-imposed restrictions and limitations of fear.
- **Black tourmaline:** Endowed with a strong healing and protective energy, it is effective in dissipating negativity and fears. It helps to maintain stability and balance the endocrine system while strengthening and revitalizing the body and mind. Its presence promotes concentration during the day and restful sleep at night, helping to relieve accumulated tensions.
- **Garnet:** It embodies courage, strength of mind, and constancy, and it is a valuable ally for those who wish to pursue their goals, also providing psychic protection against the negative energy of others.
- **Smoky quartz:** Ideal for the treatment of ailments such as headaches, colds, lower back pain, and muscle cramps, it stimulates vital energy. It can purify the root chakra, neutralize emotional excesses, and strengthen the energies needed to pursue our path.
- **Red jasper:** It is a protective and rooting gem that merges strength, vitality, and courage. Thanks to its energizing properties, it increases vigor and endurance, while acting slowly and steadily to promote healing. It encourages enthusiasm and perseverance in pursuing goals, stimulating the circulation of energy in the body.

## To Support the Second Chakra

- **The Jasper Leopard:** Works at a physical level to revitalize and teach, thus transforming our energy level. It gives power, stimulates, and awakens those who have lost their interest and passion for life, as well as victims of frozen emotions or blocked creativity. It helps to change the way of thinking and to find balance in work, attracting what you are looking for to bring harmony.
- **Orange adventuress:** It promotes enthusiasm, joy, and optimism, improving the sense of humor and giving inner balance. It is a gem that inspires creativity, ideal for artists and writers, and encourages self-forgiveness. It helps to have determination in pursuing the goals set.
- **Cornflower:** It promotes the harmony of the second chakra by bringing liveliness, centeredness, and inner peace. It transmits strong, stimulating, and creative energy, promoting a good mood and removing negativity. It can be a valuable support in the therapies for those who have suffered from physical abuse and it can help to increase sexual desire, as well as manage problems related to the menstrual cycle. It is also useful in cases of frigidity, impotence, and infertility.
- **Calcite orange:** It brings feelings of joy, optimism, and self-confidence, enhancing creativity, being also a protective gemstone that infuses energy to the physical body, stabilizes emotions, calms stress, and promotes aura regeneration. It contributes to the physical balance between male and female energies and supports the smooth functioning of the second chakra, concerning food also.

## To Support the Third Chakra

- **Citrine quartz:** It restores the solar plexus chakra's balance, enhancing confidence and personal power, as well as promoting a conscious and correct use of our energies towards others, harmonizing the chakras and promoting spontaneity, joy, hope, and a positive mentality. Free from emotional blockages and conditioning, bestowing wisdom and spiritual understanding.
- **The tiger's eye:** It offers support and is particularly suitable for those who suffer from low self-esteem and lack of creativity. Placed on the chakra of the solar plexus, it balances and releases blocked energies, making it possible to emerge and transmit our energy to others. It helps to develop self-control and establish harmony with our bodies, transmitting this sense of security to others.

- **Pyrite:** It gives a strong personal charge and energy, helping to be bright, influential, and expansive. It promotes awareness of our nature, highlighting both the positive and negative sides of a personality and promoting self-expression and personal power.
- **Yellow calcite:** It gives self-confidence and firmness, helping to face and overcome difficult situations and find the necessary energy to put ideas into practice and achieve success. It helps to overcome unbalanced reactions and emotions, promoting consistency, reliability, and self-control.
- **Amber:** It symbolizes vital energy and promotes the joy of living and awareness. It helps to dissolve and repair the negative energies accumulated in the aura, caused by stress, diseases, surgery, depression, or drug treatments, increasing the energy level and generating enthusiasm, by promoting the healing of the body, transforming negativity into positivity, and facilitating success in undertaken activities.

## To Support the Fourth Chakra

- **Malachite:** It is used to remove the negativity that afflicts the heart, giving harmony and balance to this energy center. It protects from physical dangers and negative energies, relaxing the nervous system and calming intense emotions. It also supports the resumption of spiritual evolution when interrupted by pain and despair, by helping to overcome emotional blocks that hinder well-being and personal growth.
- **Pink quartz:** Stimulates the heart's energy and is known as the gem of love. It promotes the experience of unconditional love and forgiveness towards ourselves and others, helping to overcome the fear of abandonment, and encouraging us to find love and tenderness within ourselves instead of seeking it in others.
- **Rhodochrosite:** It embodies compassion and understanding, promoting the work of our inner child and emotional well-being. It also simplifies the way to best express our feelings, being particularly addressed to those who have difficulty in showing love. It helps to let go and live with passion, encouraging optimism and developing an unconditional love to direct towards every aspect of life.
- **Chrysoprase:** It helps to not emotionally depend on others, restoring the energy balance and helping to placate negative emotions such as envy, insecurity, and tension. It brings mind strength, confidence, and inner calm, allowing us to face our daily challenges with greater security and determination.

## To Support the Fifth Chakra

- **Turquoise:** It is a gem meant to facilitate the expression of our feelings and thoughts in the calmest way possible, by healing the heart. It promotes authentic and sincere communication and is suitable for both the heart and throat chakra. This gemstone also brings protection, courage, love, friendship, money, healing, and fortune, whilst withstanding victimhood, teaching how to take control of our lives. It helps to understand and manage the root causes of events, promoting shared emotional wisdom and fostering unity among people, for positive communication between family members and individuals.
- **Blue chalcedony:** It frees from the imprisoning condition of inner silence, helping those who have difficulties expressing their needs, ideas, and emotions. It promotes a two-way kind of communication, improving our ability to listen, understand, and express ourselves and our thoughts. This gem is particularly good for those who feel confused about their emotions and opinions, encouraging an awareness of themselves and others, as well as the ability to fulfill themselves and express their desires and needs.
- **Aquamarine:** It balances the throat chakra, purifying repressed emotions and facilitating the communication of our feelings. It fosters open and authentic dialogue, even in situations of fear of judgment, while also stimulating creativity and new ideas, helping to keep calm in all circumstances.
- **The Celestine:** It is a gem aimed at promoting communication at a spiritual level, facilitating contact with the guardian angel, and bringing more awareness of the higher world. It helps us to find the way toward true awareness, supporting energy, and connection with the divine.

## To Support the Sixth Chakra

- **Amethyst:** It is highly beneficial for meditation, and it is suitable for both the sixth and seventh chakra. It fosters spiritual awareness and a deep understanding of life's events, encouraging dreams that reveal hidden truths, as well as helping to reduce anxiety and headaches, promoting mental clarity, concentration, and emotional calm. It relieves the sense of stress and emotional exhaustion, and frees from heavy emotions related to past experiences, thus facilitating the practice of meditation.
- **Lapis lazuli:** It fosters healing, joy, and psychic sensitivity, offering support and kindness, and stimulating the search for deep truths and contact with the higher self. It neutralizes the influence of the conscious mind, allowing access

to intuitive wisdom and authentic communication, promoting artistic inspiration, deep meditation, and spiritual and philosophical contemplation, as well as integrity and inner harmony.

- **Sodalite:** It is an excellent calming gem for the nervous system, and also beneficial for the throat Chakra, which helps to calm the overactive mind and give voice to our inner self, providing emotional stability and security in self-expression. It stimulates the desire for truth and knowledge, helping to develop our latent psychic potentials and to balance male and female polarities.
- **The Moonstone:** It favors intuition, femininity, and sweetness, promoting compassion and connection with our unconscious. This gem gives courage and calm, facilitating the manifestation of prophetic dreams and representing hope and purity of spirit, being particularly suitable for meditation and for the exploration of deeper, irrational aspects of life.

## To Support the Seventh Chakra

- **Hyaline quartz:** It promotes the purity of heart, feelings, and emotions, bringing clarity of mind and truth. It helps to remove energy blocks from all chakras, purifying the energy field and restoring the balance. It helps to cultivate serenity, optimism, and confidence in our life, when facing the commitments and challenges of it, by making clear the intentions of the unconscious to manifest its essence.
- **Fluorite viola:** It is also suitable for the sixth chakra and allows us to connect with the spirit, purifying the mind and facilitating lighter and cleaner thoughts. It strengthens intuition, facilitates the assimilation of new ideas, and helps to unleash our potential. It restores the energy structure of the body and aura, freeing from negative thoughts and promoting a life oriented to higher frequencies. It helps to maintain a deep connection with the earth and openness to spirituality.
- **Sugilite:** It promotes harmony with deep ideals, as well as the ability to compromise. It can also be used to purify environments, removing negativity and creating a protective light shield. It nourishes the emotional body of positivity and helps to develop psychic gifts to achieve spiritual goals, bringing peace and creativity to a mental level.
- **Selenite:** This is an extremely spiritual gem that facilitates contact with the divine. It gently dissolves harmful mental patterns, opening the mind to new perspectives and strengthening the nervous system by offering contact with guiding spirits. It also improves our telepathic abilities and guides us in the path of intro-

spection, calming confused emotional states and encouraging a more detached, objective observation of situations.

# How to Use the Gems During a Massage and More

The gems and crystals recommended by the holistic discipline can be used in various ways within the tantric context, to promote the well-being and balance of the chakras. You can use them directly during the massage, strategically placing them on the chakras' specific areas during the massage, to promote the release of blocked energies and the harmonization of energy centers. For instance, hyaline quartz could be placed on the seventh chakra, whilst violet fluorite could be used for the sixth.

The gems can also be heated and used, promoting muscle relaxation and opening the energy channels. Indeed, during the massage, hot gemstones can be used to stimulate specific points of the chakras and promote the circulation of vital energy.

Another way to employ them is through guided meditation, before or after the massage, where you can guide the receiver to a guided meditation using the recommended gems for the specific chakras, which can help you consolidate the effects of the practice and promote greater energy awareness. The stones can also be used in ceremonies of purification and harmonization of the environment, which can help create a sacred space and foster a deeper connection with vital energy during treatment.

In addition to that, personalized treatments can be made too, since each person has unique energy needs and the singular gems can be chosen according to the specific demands of the receivers. The holistic therapist can recommend specific gemstones based on the treatment goals and individual energy challenges of the other.

Anyway, let's not forget that the gems can also be used to decorate our massage temple, being placed around the futon on the floor or on a shelf.

In general, the use of recommended gems in the holistic discipline within a tantra massage aims at promoting the release of physical and emotional tensions, as well as promoting energy balance and supporting the general well-being of the receiver.

Here, we have offered you detailed information on oils and gems that, although it is not mandatory for you to follow, can greatly enrich your tantric experience. This insight is designed for those who wish to enrich their practice by following holistic notions, for not only do gems and oils promote physical well-being but they also stimulate the senses both spiritually and sensorially.

At the same time, essential oils offer a fragrance that influences the sense of smell, as well as promotes relaxation and emotional harmony. It is important to reiterate that there is no obligation in the use of these resources, but they offer an *opportunity* to deepen the practice and enrich the overall experience. The main purpose is to focus and visualize the treatment of individual chakras through the use of gems and corresponding oils, promoting a holistic sense of well-being and a deeper connection with body and spirit.

# 4. Pave The Way: The Tantric Massage as a Preparation for Yoni Experience

Once you have carefully prepared your massage temple, it is fundamental for you to welcome the receiver in a comfortable and respectful environment. This is the reason why it is advisable to perform the treatment while completely naked, to promote a deep connection with the body and the vital energy. However, it is crucial to respect the comfort and individual preferences of both participants, since the other person may wish to start the procedure by wearing a sarong or a scarf to cover their intimate parts, which is to be respected. It is also important to create a safe and non-judgmental space where people can feel free to express their needs and preferences, and as time passes and the massage starts, the receiver might start to feel more and more comfortable and decide to finally take it all off.

To create the perfect environment for your tantric massage, follow these three keys that will help you practice it with yourself before anyone else and get ready before starting:

**The first key is spiritual presence**, which requires both participants to agree and be fully present and aware, willing to participate in the procedures. If you feel any kind of resistance or doubt, it is better to *stop*. Being present means looking into the other person's eyes, giving the other away and understanding if they are laughing or crying, keeping eye contact, and nodding to let them know you are there to support them and give them nothing else but love.

**The second key is related to conscious breathing.** Invite the receiver to breathe using the mouth, accompanying the act of exhalation with a sound of liberation, so as for their body to open up and fully enjoy the pleasure.

**The third key is the conscious touch.** During the massage, focus on the part of the body you are touching, imagining cleaning and purifying it, and avoid getting distracted in any way, but stay focused on your partner.

By following these three keys during your tantric massage, you will be able to perform a professional massage accurately and consciously!

# Calm Your Body and Mind Through Breathing and Meditation

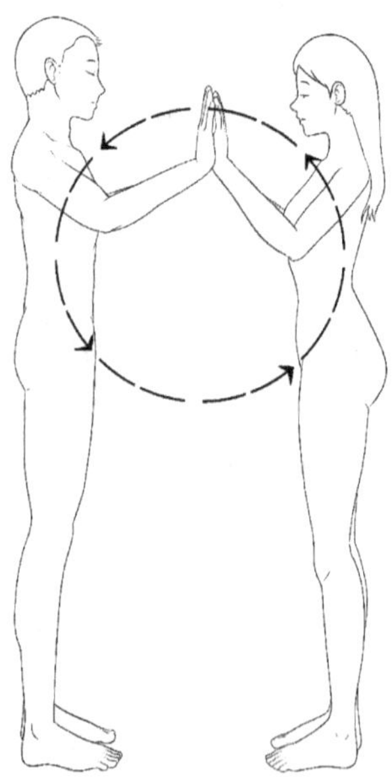

*Shared Breathing*

Before starting the massage, it is essential to get your mind and body fully ready through deep breathing cycles, which do not just help you to calm your psyche, but also pave the way for a deeper and more conscious connection during the treatment.

Stay on the track of a deep and regular kind of breathing, to create a relaxing sound while exhaling. You should start breathing by focusing on the first chakra and then gradually rise to the other ones, up to the seventh. Also, keep breathing synchrony during this cycle.

**Afterward, you can practice a shared kind of breathing, sitting, or also standing, in front of your partner and intertwining your hands. As the man is inhaling with his nose, he must place his hands together with the woman's on his heart and, as he exhales, he must drop his hands along with his breath to his first chakra, touching it slightly. At the same time, as the woman is inhaling and the man exhaling, holding his hands over his Yoni, energy will be transferred into her body, penetrating it through Yoni, which will cross her body and then leave from the heart.**

This sets up a cycle of shared energy and breathing, where the male pole connects with the female's, creating a powerful exchange of energies and a deep connection between the two. Intertwined hands symbolize the energy flow that moves through both chakras, creating a harmonious union between the male and female poles. During this process, the massage giver starts their inspiration from the heart, then passes through the lower chakras and then exhales from the first one, while the receiver inhales from their first chakra and then passes through the other ones to the first one, and exhales from the heart chakra. This flow of energy expands through the body of the receiver and goes up to the heart, the point from which the woman exhales while the giver inhales, and so forth and so on. Repeat this exercise as many times as you think is best for you to feel ready.

The man, at the moment of the woman's exhalation, receives this energy in his heart and guides it through his chakras, allowing a flow of harmonious and shared energy, while also creating an energetic dance between the two, merging their vital flows into a single powerful one. This way, the breathing cycle becomes a form of deep energetic communication and a tangible manifestation of the union between the male and female poles. During the practice, the woman needs to keep in mind the male energy always (*Shiva*), as it penetrates into her (*Shakti*). By imagining this exchange of energy and love, we can promote a deeper connection and greater awareness of our flowing, all this through the union act of the hands, as a preparatory phase.

# A Step-by-Step Guide to Preparatory Sensual Tantra Massage

As we keep in mind that Yoni is the first chakra and that during our massage session, we must also take into account all of the other six, the tantric massage represents, by convention, a sort of preparation to Yoni, since **we perform a kind of massage involving the whole body, guiding the flow of energy from the bottom up, and then descending in a circular and sinuous movement, as if it were a dance.** This movement aims at following the path of kundalini energy, which is pretty similar to the movement of a snake when crawling.

During the massage, we must focus and accompany this energy, being fully present in the moment and focused on giving love and benefits to the other, while also contemplating the woman's body as a way to rebalance the respective energies, show affection, and focus on bringing benefit and freeing the other from any kind of negativity, that is the main purpose. At this stage, the woman must let herself go and abandon any form of control, trusting her partner while relaxing and fully enjoying the treatment.

Only this way is it possible to open up to an authentic kind of pleasure, reaching a kind of ecstasy that would normally seem unattainable. **This ritual can produce a deep sense of relaxation, while simultaneously igniting a flame of burning desire working on the mind and body and preparing the woman to receive.**

In addition to this, the sensual massage sharpens our sense of awareness, making it possible to explore our being more deeply, by also embracing our femininity and masculinity with greater intensity. It is an instinctive art, performed without rules and only guided by a burning desire to bring pleasure to your beloved. Caresses, stroking, gentle hand movements, and intertwining fingers create a natural, unprecedented flow of love, without borders or patterns.

I suggest dedicating at least 50 minutes, or even 60, to this act to ensure a complete openness to the bliss of pleasure. Without this preparatory act, the receiver may struggle to completely let go of their control, limiting the depth of pleasure that Yoni can give.

In the initial phase, we can also expand the relaxation state through a massage on the whole body. Starting with one finger, then adding more until using both hands for both light and deep strokes, remember **the total presence in the gesture, the focusing of energy, and the visualization of our body as a tool for energy rebalancing.**

Hands must almost touch the skin, especially when moving from the top to the bottom, for a more decisive pressure to be applied on the opposite movement. This way, we can use both of the energy flows present in our being, Shakti and Shiva. The latter, the male one as we rise and apply more pressure, and the first, the female one when our hands are coming down from above, letting it flow, be guided, and receive the pleasure.

The massage giver should keep a deep state of breathing, in sync with the receiver's breath, more relaxed, and contrary to the breathing of the preparation phase; the giver must follow and synchronize their breath with the receiver, continuing to share the cycles (when the receiver inhales, the giver inhale, and vice versa). **In this state of energy exchange, we do not simply massage the woman's body, but we are allowing ours to be massaged by hers too, creating a deep connection that goes beyond mere words!**

Although it might look quite complex, this tantric practice has been studied and practiced for centuries in the East, and through its understanding, we can access a deeper level of connection and pleasure. Indeed, even though it is a free form of art, it is useful to learn the basic movement sequence to take control of the situation with confidence.

Here is a series of simple steps to follow to get an infinite set of variations, according to your personal preferences. Usually, it is suggested to start by massaging the other person while they are in a prone position or on their stomach, and then proceed to the supine position for a deeper immersion in the initial relaxation.

Tantra massage can be divided into five phases plus one (five times equal five positions plus one), three of which require the prone position of the receiver and the supine one of the giver, going on then with a sixth phase, the specific one for Yoni and that still requires the supine position, always.

Who is in charge of performing the massage must be on their knees and move around the body to be massaged, as a way to contemplate it.

Below is the "cycle of tantra massage" in perfect sequence (from one to five), to achieve a full flow of energies. After the fifth phase, you can start the Yoni massage by standing between the open legs of the receiver in a supine position, kneeling, or also in a more comfortable position in front of Yoni.

Below is the sense of energy that flows to the body and the complete cycle of the preparatory massage, whilst in the next chapter, we will tackle a deeper Yoni massage description.

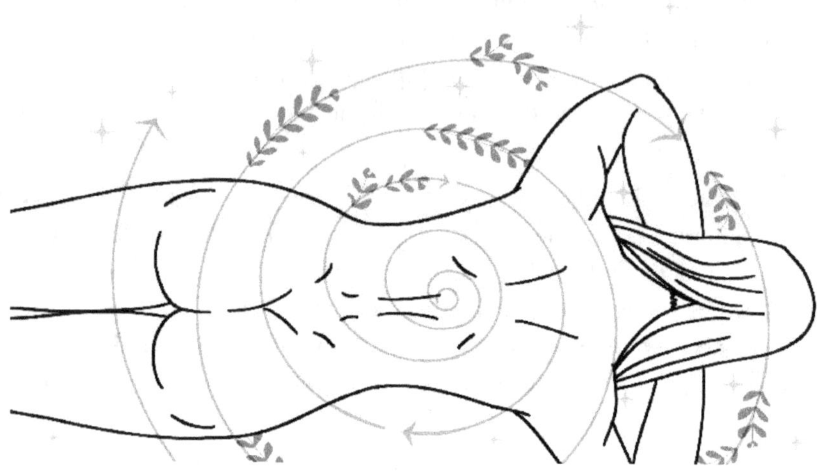

*Imagine a flow of energy running through your body*

## THE CYCLE OF TANTRA MASSAGE

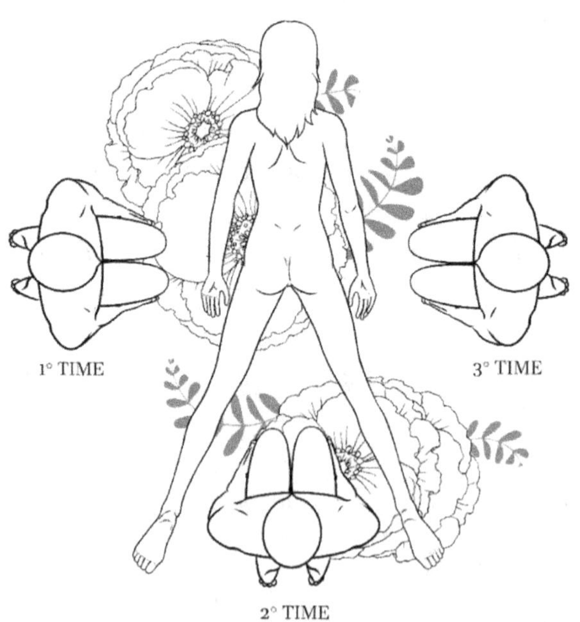



*First three phases with her in prone position*

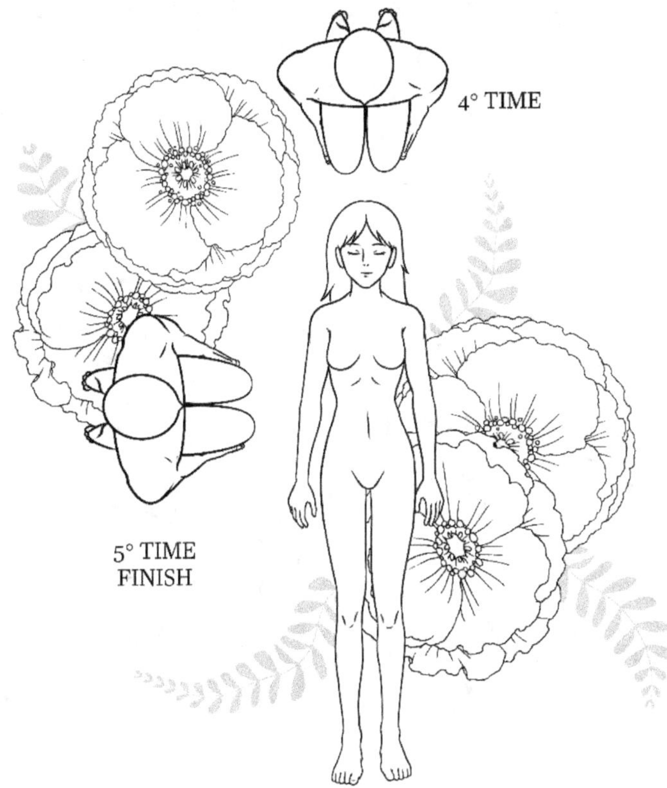

*Next two phases with her in supine position*

Whenever you switch off your position, always do it with an initial tantric touch starting from the heart and going towards the lower extremities, then going up again to the crown, as shown in the image.

Follow the same path as the signals below. **Image A represents the initial path, to be repeated three times each time you change your position. Keep that in mind.**

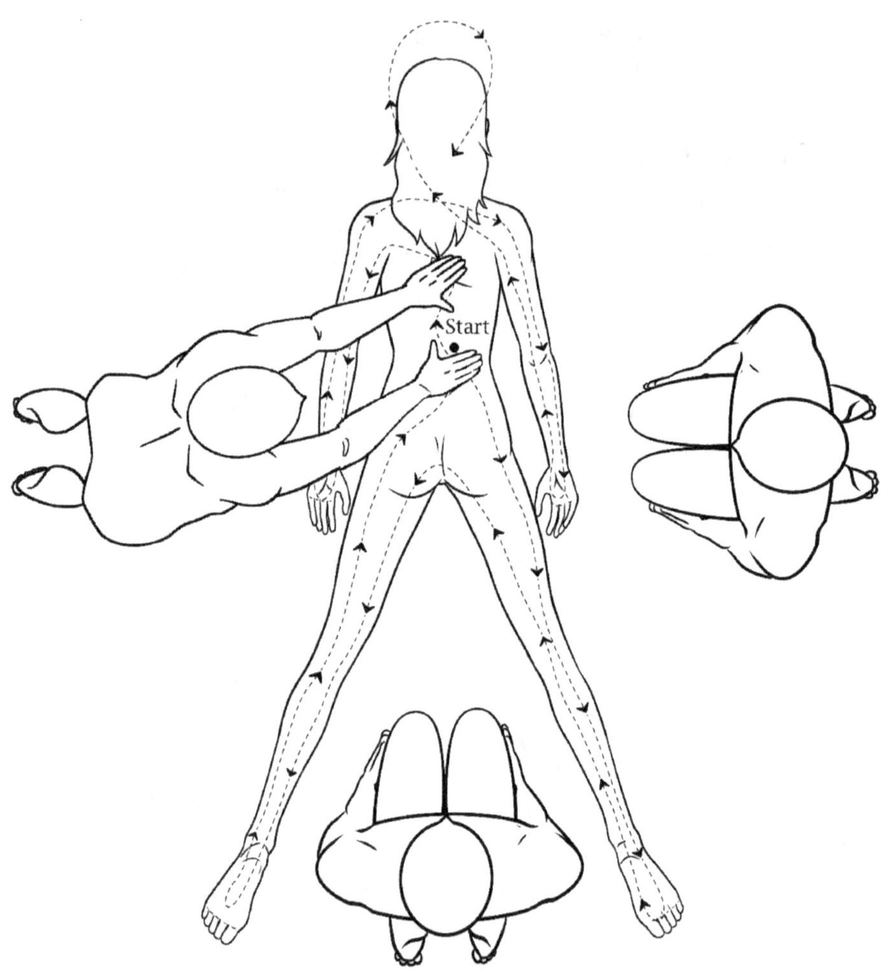

**Image A.** *Massage path that remains unchanged every time you change the position (repeated 3 times), even when the receiver is in a supine position, covering all 5 positions*

## 1 TIME: Position 1

Once you have prepared the environment and the woman is sitting in the room (or in any other place), and after you have shared your breathing cycles, as explained above, invite her to lie down in a prone position on the futon as you kneel on your left side. Place your left hand on her back, near the heart (the fourth chakra, or heart chakra, according to Hinduism and Buddhism is the meeting point between the body and the spirit) and the right hand in the back, as in the image below (second chakra, also known as the sacral chakra, is located just below the navel, in the lower part of the abdomen, and because of its position is our "center," the core of emotional energy).

Try to always stay in contact with her body, at least with one hand, keep this in mind when you change positions. The touch must be light, Tantric Touch, now try to synchronize your breathing with hers, stay synchronized and still for 30 seconds, get rid of all worries and concentrate on her who should feel relieved by your presence. The human body is also energy, let's imagine this energy moving clockwise along the body, see this energy, imagine seeing it, it is this energy that now needs to be channeled, balanced, purified from all negativity, it is time to be one with your partner, and it will be your massage, your energy that will accompany her rebalancing, while you are in contact with her, concentrate on the visualization of your spirituality and your energy, you are concentrated only on her, imagine sweeping away her negativity, simulate, every now and then, while you caress, sweeping away with your hands as if you were dusting them off the body and at the same time visualize the negativity that is being chased away.

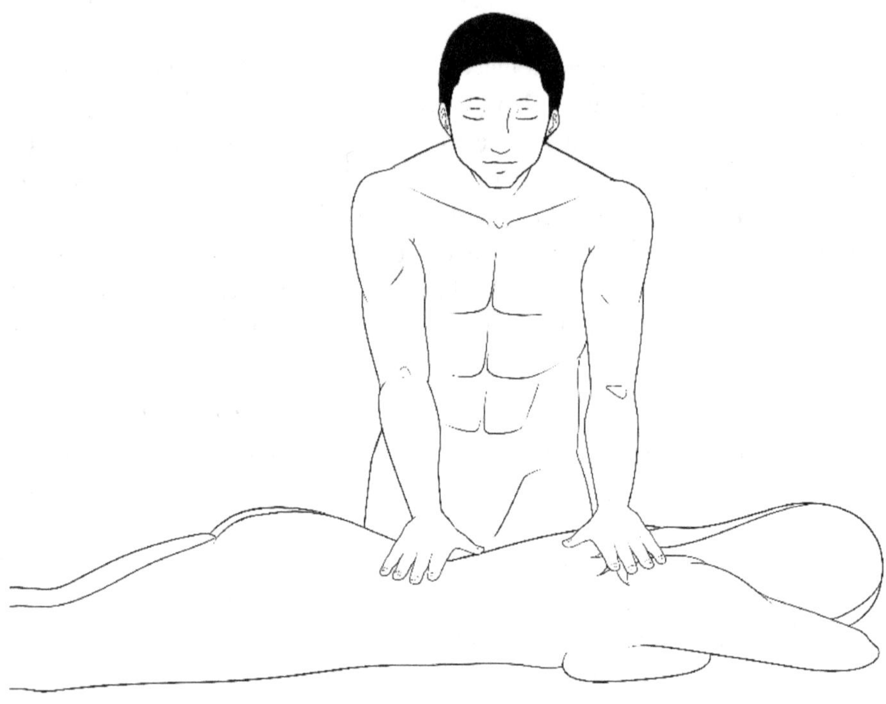

*Start position, hands on the second and fourth chakra.*

## Position 2

With your hands resting on her second and fourth chakra (position 1), make circular movements in a clockwise direction, as if to make her body perceive your presence. **Then start to stroke her with both hands, following the flow of the path traced in *Image A*,** previously shown.

To make it all even more sensual and delicate, you could start to caress her whole body, with only one finger also, adding another finger as you go on until both hands are used. Below, the whole massage route is described in this position of *Image A* (to be repeated three times). You will need to repeat the same procedure every time you switch your position; from now on, this will be *implied* and *will not be repeated.*

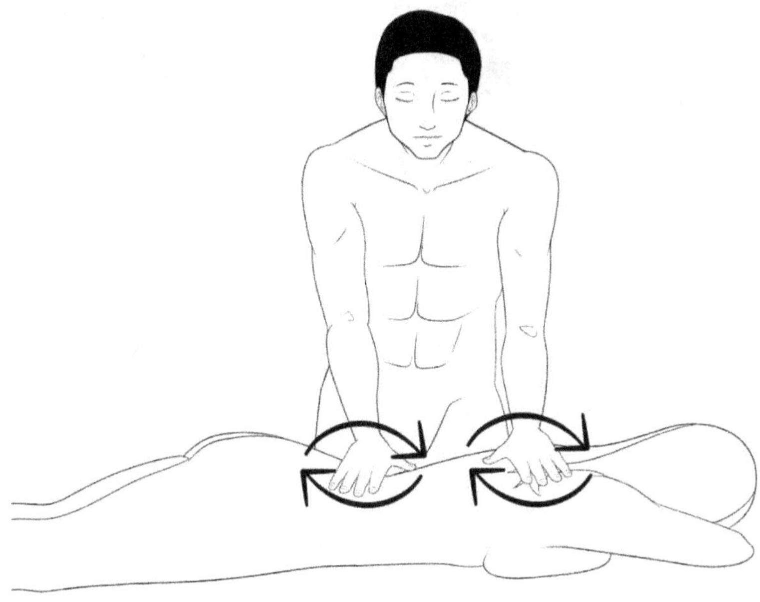

*Three simultaneous circular movements, with your hands on the second and fourth chakra.*

## Position 3

After having made the three circles, starting from the starting position, at the same time slide the palms of your hands with a very light touch, almost touching it, from the starting point of position 1-2, up to the right foot passing through the leg with a continuous and constant movement, when you reach the bottom perform a grip with pressure under the heel in the opposite direction, as if to push the energy towards the head, then go up the leg always with a sinuous caress trying to use both hands (with one you massage the outside thigh, with the other the inside), up to her buttocks, caress them and then go back down on the left leg, doing the same, remember, when you go up, while you pass over the buttocks, slide the little finger in the middle (figure M), touching her intimacy, so that you will cause her a shiver of pleasure and the beginning of the sensation of awakening of the senses.

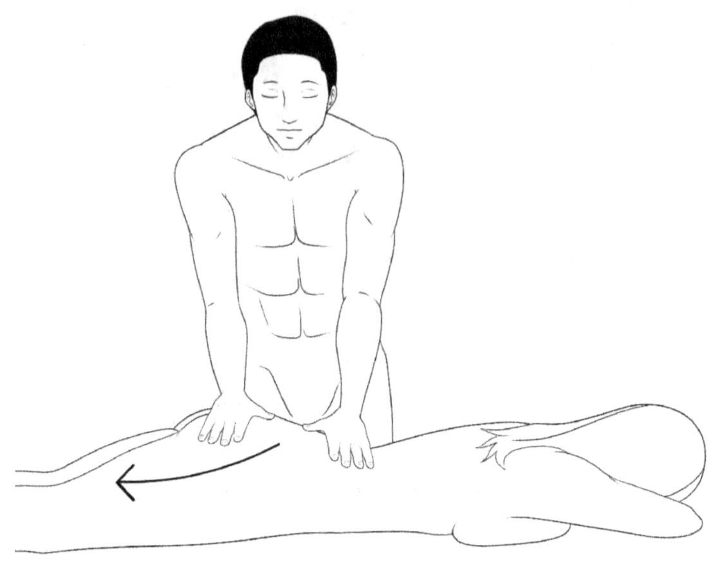

*Start the massage following the path illustrated in Image A*

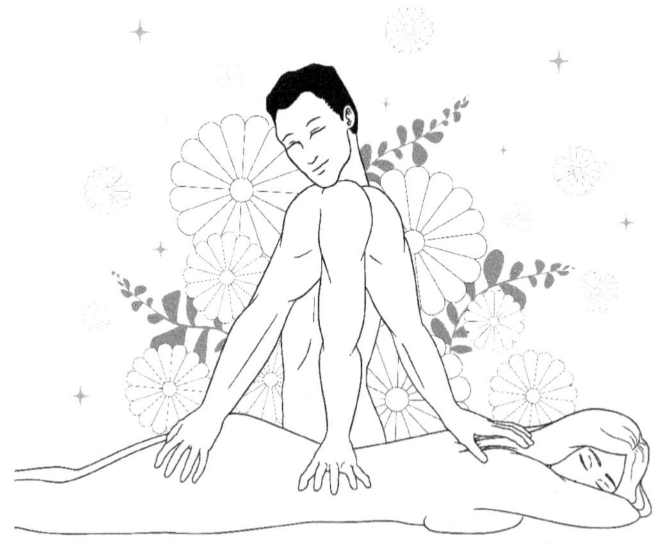

*Caress the whole body with both hands, from top to bottom and vice versa following the path of image A.*

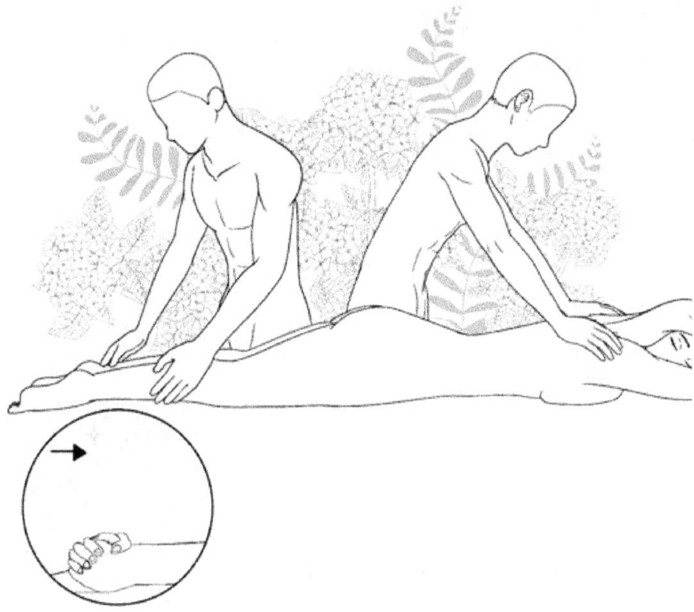

*Grab her heel and push up firmly.*

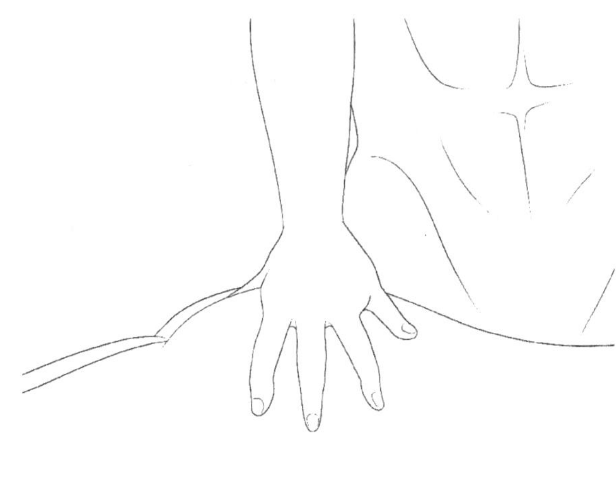

**Image M.** *The little finger touches the Yoni every time it rises with the massage.*

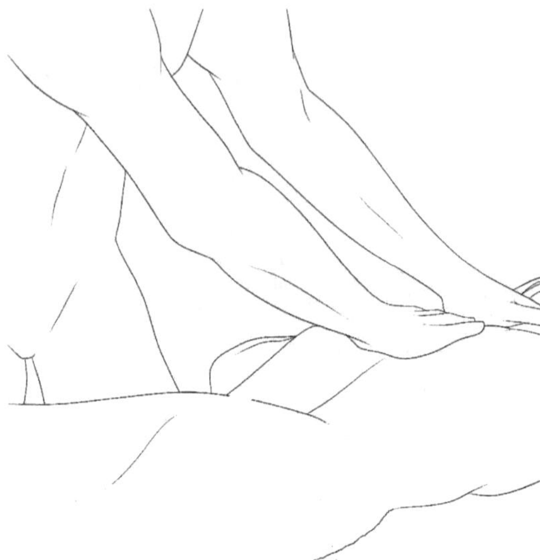

*Massage from bottom to top, following the path shown in image A.*

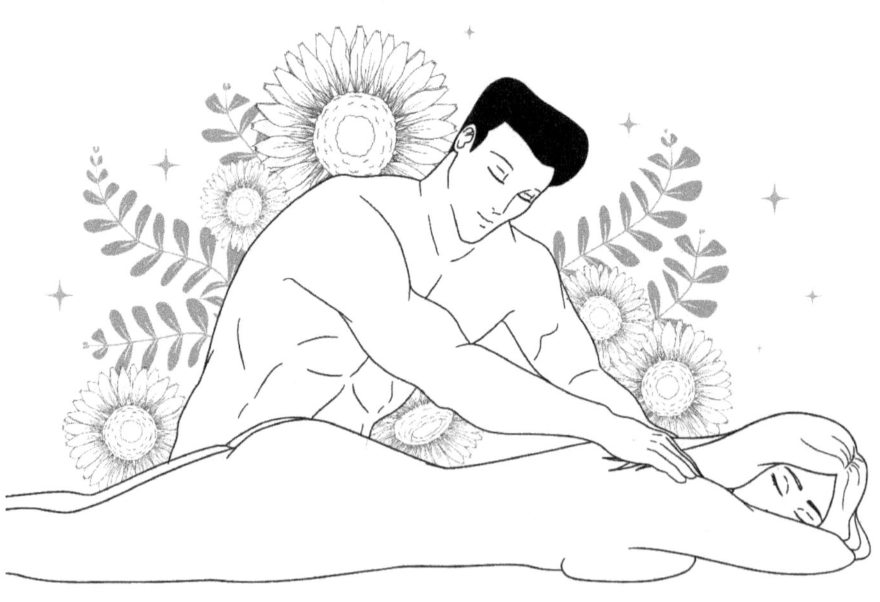

*Full body massage with two hands.*

## Position 4

Now, go upwards from the buttocks, towards the back, and then go down from the left arm side, stroking it until the hand. Touch it with a little more pressure, then raise your arm and do the same with the other one. Touch the crown, imagine getting energy from the seventh chakra (which connects us with the universal energy and through which we can reach the light of knowledge and awareness of our being, serenity, and perception of unity in the whole), and balance it with other energy points.

Perform this from the bottom up and down, remembering that, every time you climb, the "curious" little finger touches the first chakra in the middle of the buttocks, and every time you descend to the feet, it makes a slight squeeze with an upward pressure.

Perform these cycles slowly and gently, at least three times, taking all the time to contemplate the body, purify the energy, and elevate the spirit. Then, bend your body over her so as for your chest to rest slightly on her back and make it fit together. Align your chakras, place your arms as if to embrace her, bring your head closer to hers, let your bodies touch, and swing slightly as if to rock her, with no hurry, but just keep her in your arms.

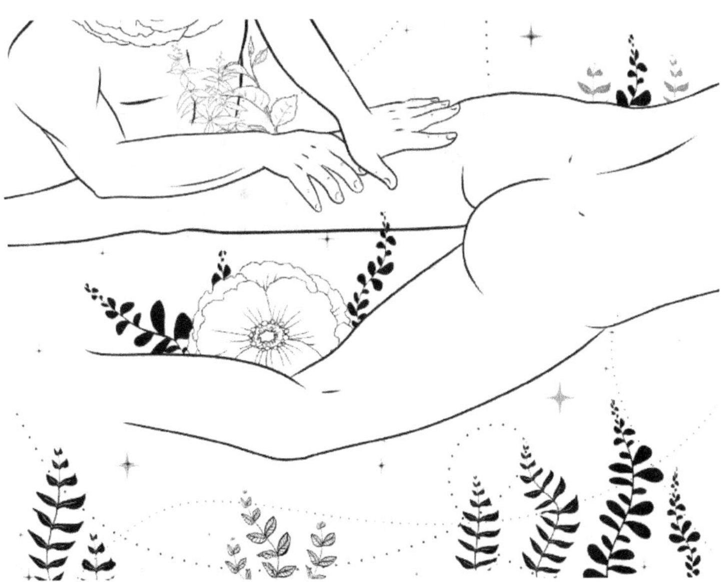

*Full body massage with two hands.*

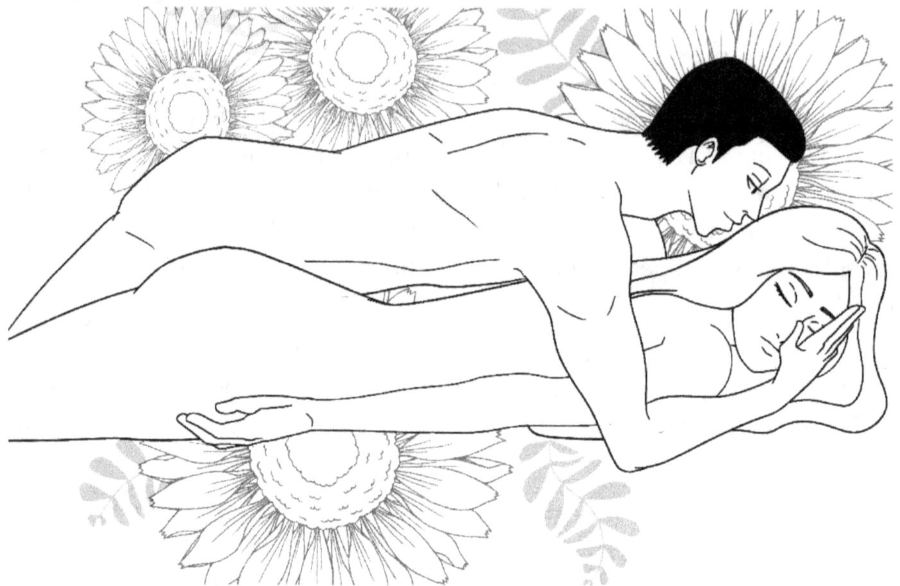

*Hug, gentle swinging and chakra alignment.*

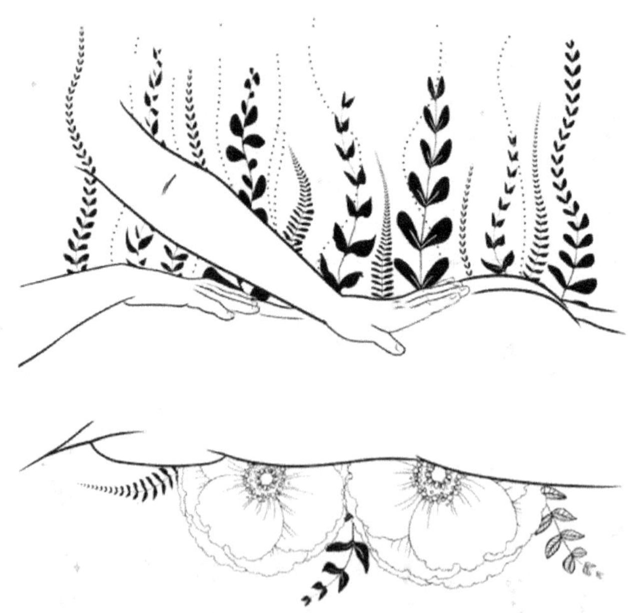

*Massage all over the body always following the direction of the arrows in image A.*

## 2 TIME: Position 5–6

After hugging her, return to the starting position and continue to caress her freely and instinctively. Next, place your left hand on her second Chakra and, using it as a support point, quickly change position without removing your hand. Enter between her legs, first inserting a knee right between them. While you do this, with both hands (so the left one detaches from her sacrum, the second Chakra), delicately caress her legs, sliding softly from her buttocks to her feet. Then, with a firm gesture, grab her ankles and spread her legs, entering the position under her with the other knee as well. Now you are between her legs (2 TIME).

It is very important that this movement of spreading the legs once you have grabbed the ankles, is very sudden and decisive, because it causes a very exciting sensation, putting you in front of the first Chakra (It is located between the genitals and the anus, its element is the earth and the symbol is the square, it is connected to the adrenal glands, the large intestine and the skeletal system). Every time you change position, first of all, caress the whole body with 3 repeated cycles as shown previously (following the path of image A), always in a clockwise direction, passing the palms of the hands along the whole body. For convenience, if you want, you can also put a hand on the futon to lean on and lift yourself up on your legs so as to also touch above the head, you must feel comfortable, at ease and relaxed, transmitting the same to the receiver, take care of her, her body, her soul and her chakras.

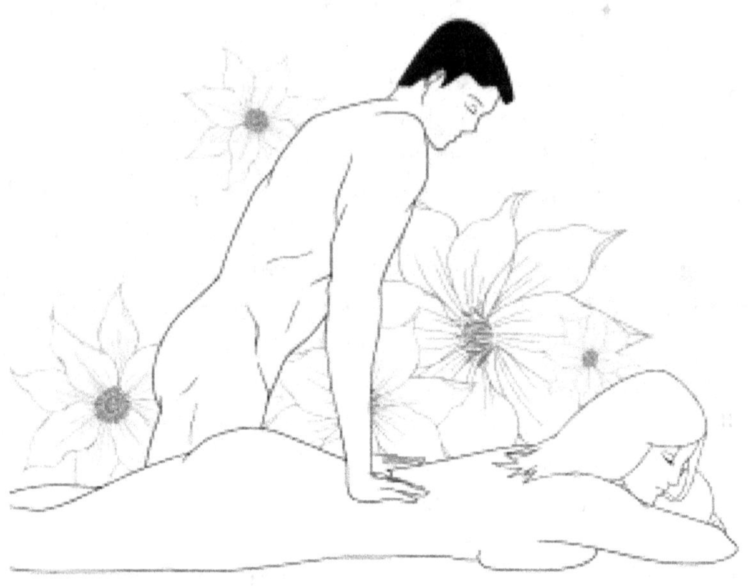

*Change of position via lever on the receiver*

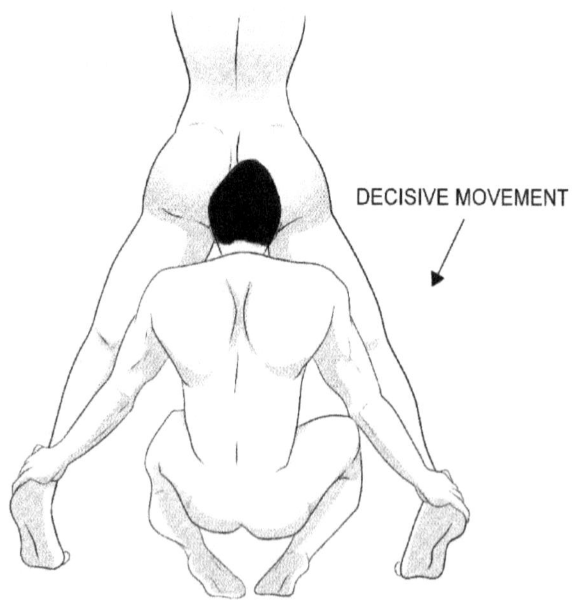


*Grab the ankles and spread them with a decisive movement.*

## Position 7

Whenever you change your position, remember to first of all caress her whole body, always following the clockwise movement of *Image A*. Stop on her main energy points, while giving all that you have in the massage, letting go of every kind of bad energy and putting all of your emotions, passion, feelings, and creativity. Focus on the area around the first and second chakras, continuing with a clockwise motion while also exploring the other upper chakras.

Then, take a silk scarf and let it slide over her body, passing it along her back until it gently touches her buttocks and legs. Play with it and use your imagination, to fully enjoy this pleasant and exciting experience! **The scarf is the perfect representation of the tantric touch. Always keep in mind the importance of putting tenderness and delicacy in all of your touches, just as a soft silk fabric.** While playing with it, let it slide along her buttocks as if to seek her intimacy with a gentle gesture.

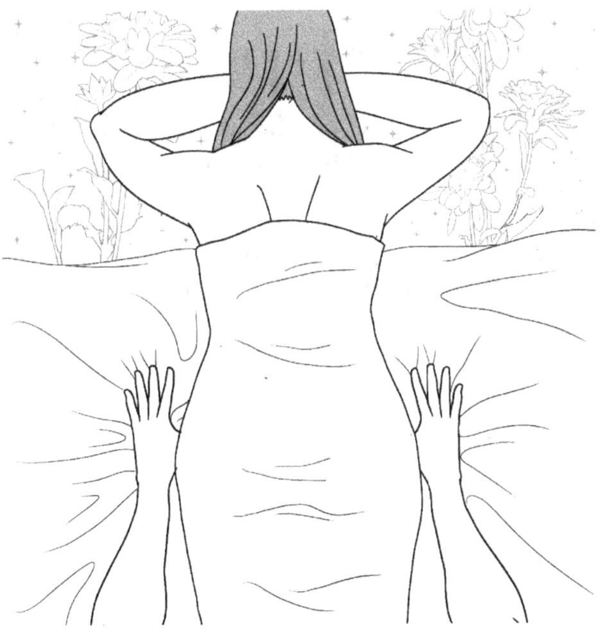

*Caress using a scarf.*

## Position 8

The moment of the use of the oil brings us closer to her first chakra, to her intimacy, and her pleasure. Even though before arriving at this moment you have already approached her Yoni with your little finger only, it is only thanks to the oil that you can really come into contact with her intimacy. Here's how:

Place your left hand in a position to shape a spoon, and place it right above her pubic area, without touching it yet; gently pour hot oil over it and hold it in your hand. Free your right hand and open your left one slightly so as for the oil to slide down between your fingers on her bottom and down to her Yoni.

Place your right hand under all this and move the knuckles of your right hand, gently touching her lips to start lubricating them. **The oil sensation together with the hand movement will provoke a revival of her sexual energy.** Practice this massage with a movement of the knuckles from top to bottom and vice versa, while stroking her first chakra. Imagine the knuckles' movement as if they were the keys of a piano.

In the meanwhile, caress her buttocks using your left hand, to activate, free, and awaken her second chakra (*sexual energy*). Continue massaging the lower back and inner thigh, remaining close to Yoni. Get acquainted with her pleasure as the energy starts to wake up. Do everything slowly, making sure that your hands are full of oil.

In the image below, the knuckles are all aligned and are moving like the keys of a piano, creating a very pleasant massaging effect that will surely start to excite her.

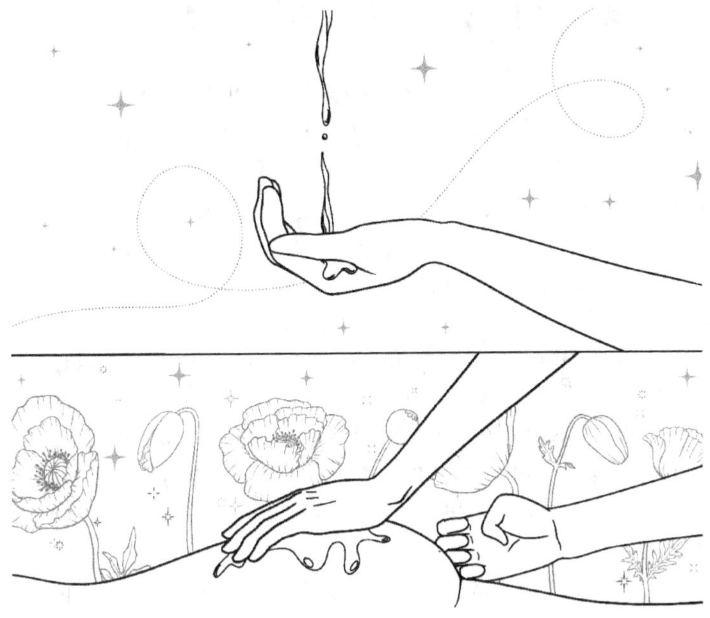

*Pour the oil out on your left hand and let it softly fall on Yoni.*

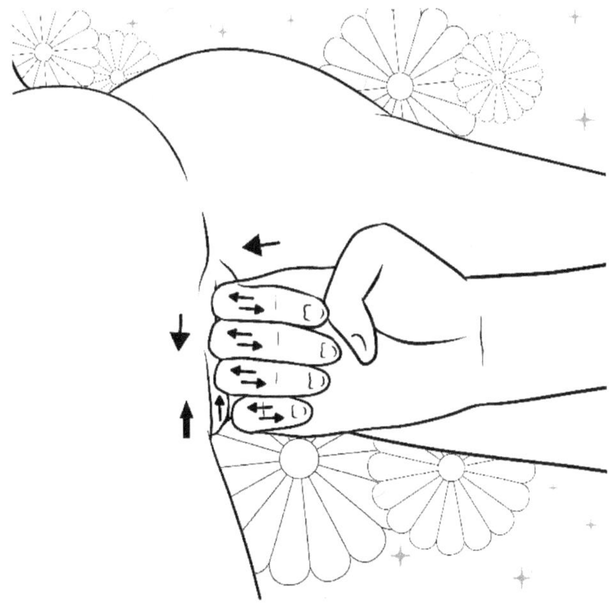

*Knuckles massage with piano-like movements, top-down, and vice versa*

## Position 9

You can choose which hand to use based on your comfort: if you are right-handed, you will probably be more comfortable with your right hand. At this stage, I remind you, you are kneeling behind her, between her legs.

After awakening the sexual energy in her, guide this energy towards her heart, her throat and finally her crown. Massage gently with both hands, in a wavy motion, to bring this sexual energy up from her first Chakra to the seventh. Use your hands as a convoy to rebalance this energy, following a fluid movement similar to that of a snake slithering upwards (Kundalini). It is as if her Kundalini energy is flowing, nourishing all the other energy points along its path. With each touch, allow this energy to ascend, bringing harmony and balance to her entire being. To reach her head, you may need to support yourself with the other hand; so, you will hardly be able to massage with both hands at the same time, you will need one to rest on the ground.

However, there is no prohibition in lifting yourself up with your legs, as if you were doing squats, to reach her. During this process, try to caress her entire body, including her extremities. If necessary, temporarily change position, going from kneeling to bending over your legs. Feel free to move as you see fit, to explore her entire temple. The indications are basic principles, then you should do your part, following her breathing and your sensations.

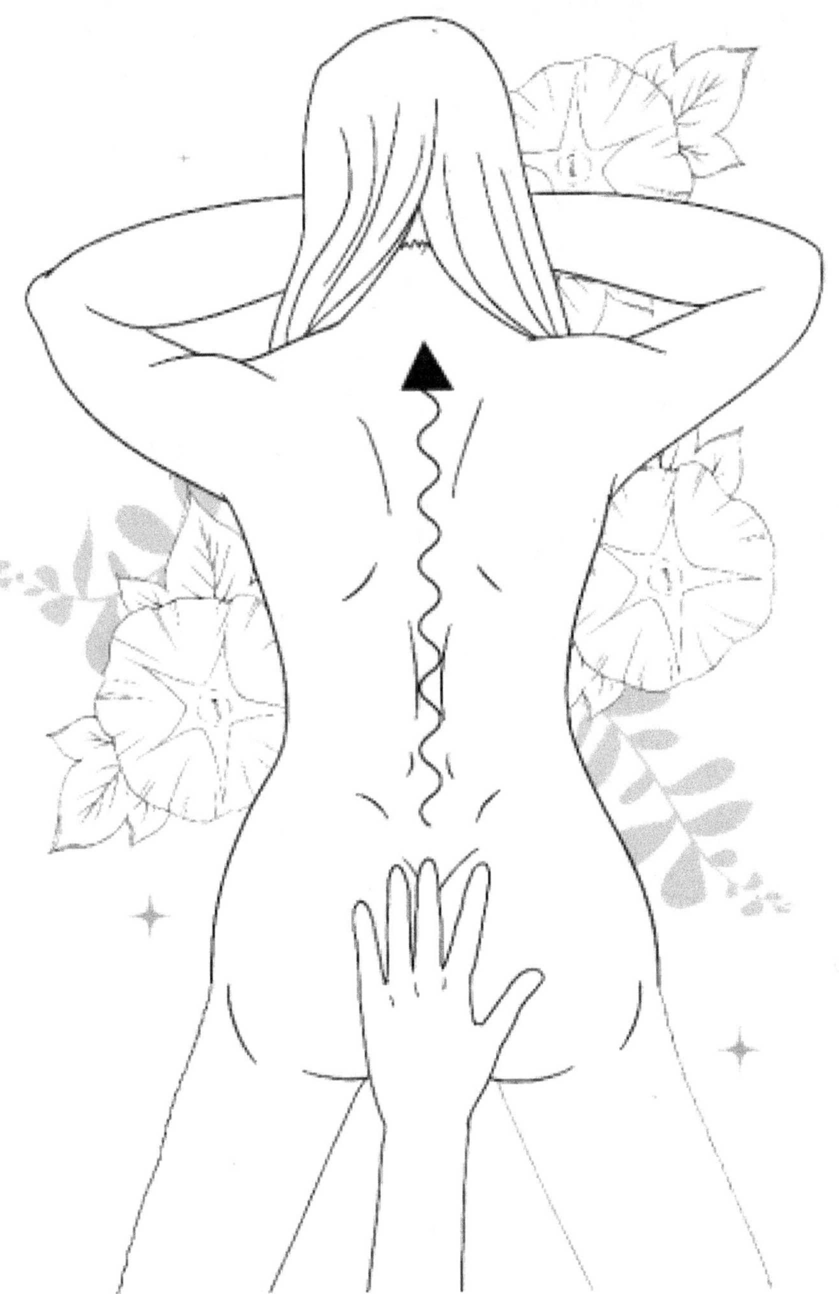

*Wavy massage from bottom to top*

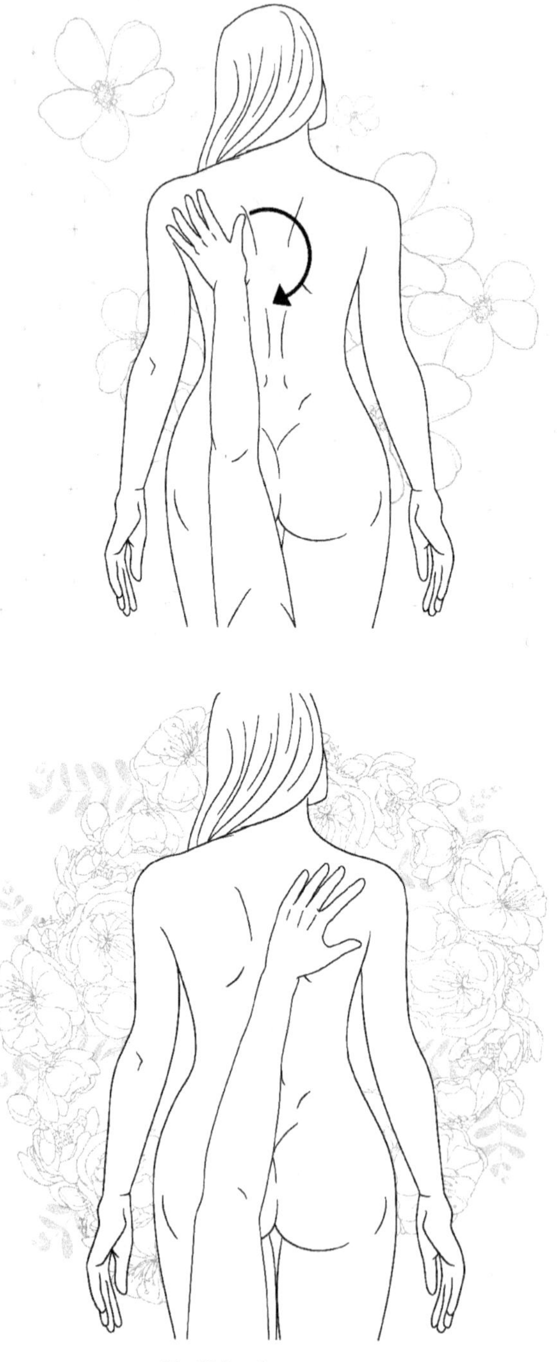

*Full body massage.*

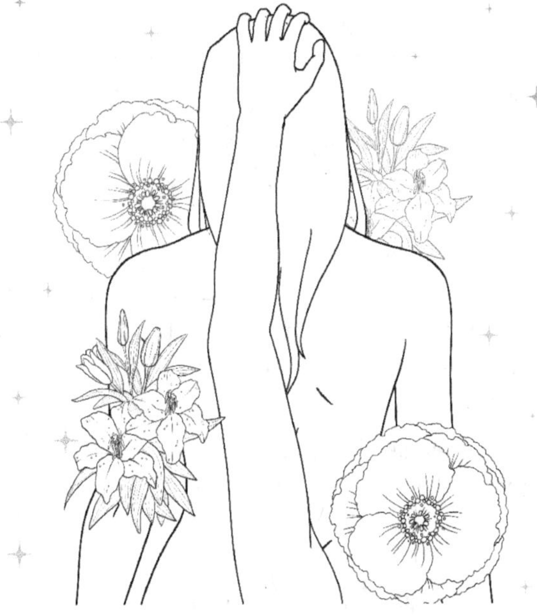

*Crown massage.*

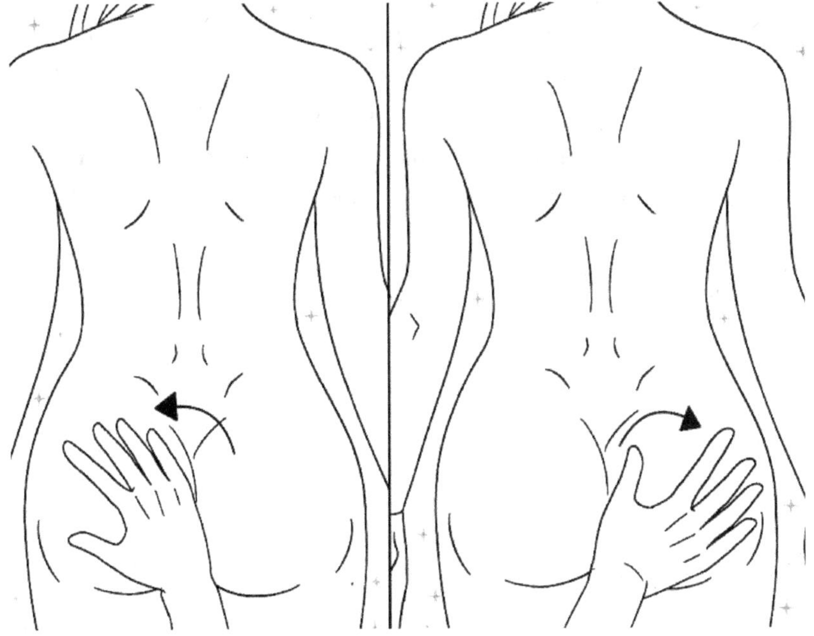

*Full body massage including buttocks.*

## Position 10

This step is essential because it establishes the first real contact between your hand and her first Chakra.

Place your right hand open at 90 degrees from the floor, with your arm almost resting on the futon, at knee height and slide it gently towards her Yoni, caressing the inside of her thigh until you come into contact with it, focusing on her first Chakra and connecting with her sexual energy. Still with your hand open, apply light pressure on the Yoni and make it vibrate, and stay for about twenty seconds, feel her Yoni, breathe with it, then move that hand and the other along her back, following the central axis with a wavy movement similar to that of a snake. Repeat this process three times.

During this movement, you take her energy from the first Chakra and accompany it, rebalancing all the other points along the central axis of her back. It is as if you were embracing all her energy points, bringing harmony and balance. As you go up, focus on all the other Chakras, up to the crown, do not rush. Then, go back down and repeat the movement, that is, with the right hand still open at 90 degrees to the ground, with the arm almost resting on the futon at knee height, slide gently towards your Yoni, caressing the inner thigh until contact, stay on it, apply light pressure and make it vibrate, but this time, instead of going up on the back, go up on the right buttock with a circular motion, clockwise, then go back to the inner thigh and repeat the movement three times, then do the same on the left buttock.

This process helps to stimulate and harmonize the energy throughout your body, allowing you to connect more deeply with yourself and with your first Chakra.

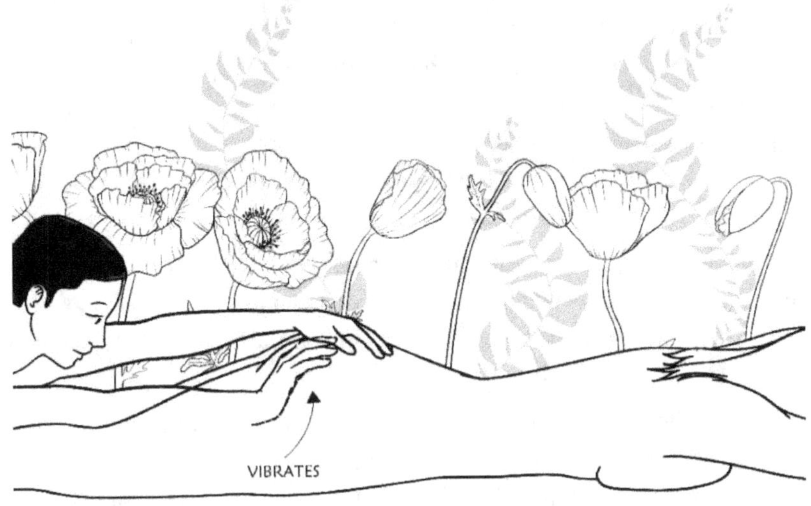



*Open palm movement vibrating continuously in pressure on the Yoni, while with the other hand performing a massage on the second Chakra.*

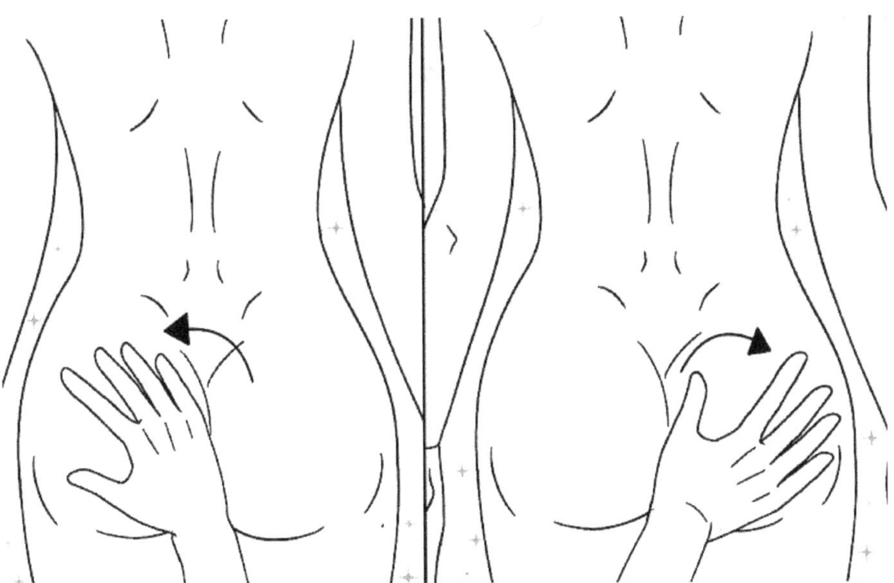

*Hand in support and vibrating on the Yoni and massage on the right buttock and then the left.*

## Position 11

Now go back to stimulating her Yoni with your knuckles as explained before, from top to bottom to stimulate the first Chakra, then when you bring your hand down, shape it into a spoon and place it under her pubic area touching it, stay still for a few seconds and come into contact with her energy. With the other hand, massage her lower back and back (Second, Third and Fourth Chakra).

Next, stimulate and massage with your fingertips with a delicate movement giving light taps, as if you were playing a piano, the fingers move up and down, and alternate with a circular movement caressing the clitoris and the labia and playing with them a little, while with the thumb you stimulate the perineum.

Go up to bring the energy to her back and then go down caressing her legs. Repeat three times. To caress her legs, always remain kneeling between her legs and, at the same time with both arms, bring them back as far as you can. From the feet, go up, caressing the inside of the thighs until you touch her private parts. In the image I show the left hand that stimulates her vagina and with the other one caresses the upper energy points, but if you are more comfortable you can also invert the hands at this point.

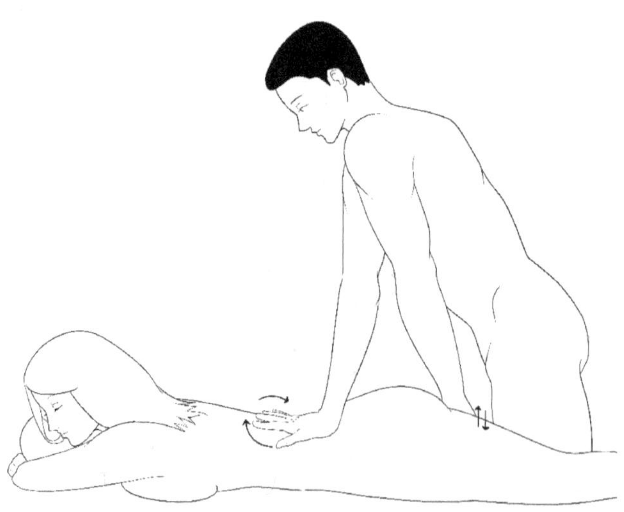

*Simultaneous massage of the Yoni and the upper Chakras.*

## Position 12

After taking care of her chakras and stimulating the most intimate parts, lie down and hug her, to align your chakras to hers and synchronize your breath. Then, gently switch position.

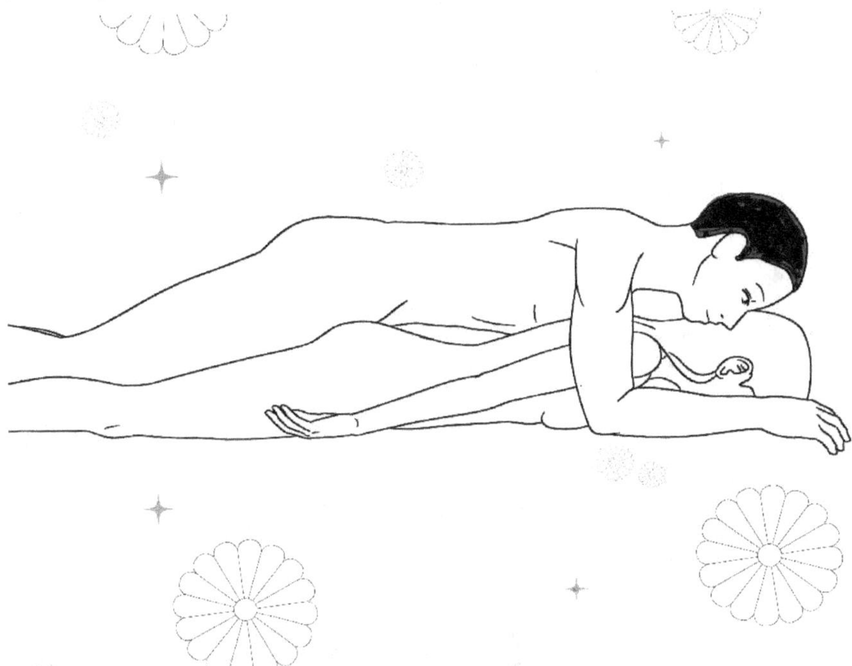

*Hug before changing positions.*

## 3 TIME: Position 13

Hold your hand on the second chakra and move to the right side, always kneeling at her side. Stroke her whole body as you do every time you change positions, following the image. Imagine throwing away all negativity, feeling happy as you caress her whole body and transmit your feelings, as well as your desire to take care of her.

After massaging, stroke her with your left hand, bottom-top, and then with your right hand, top-bottom, so that the sexual energy meets the heart at the center of the receiver's back. Visualize the rebalancing of her chakras and the elimination of energy blocks and negativity.

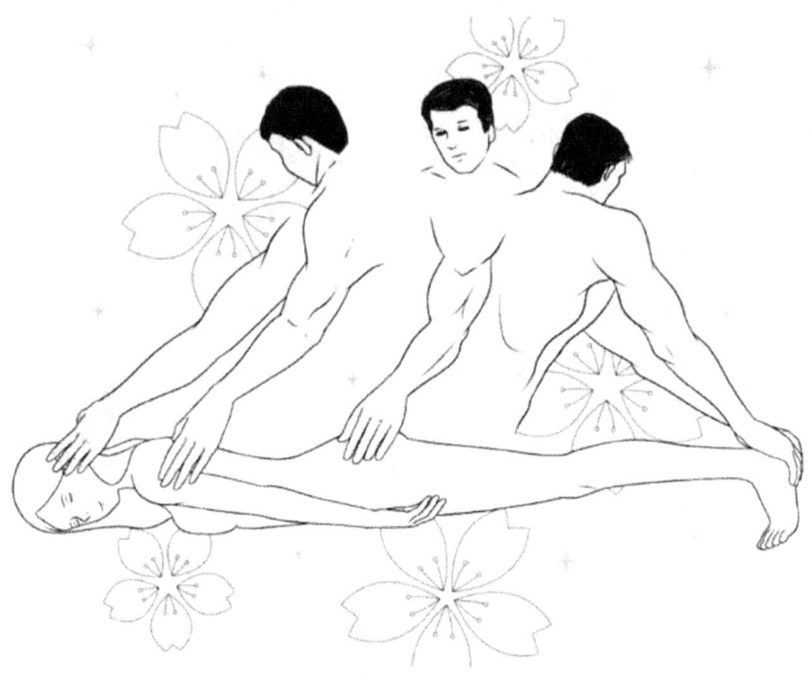

*Whole body massage.*

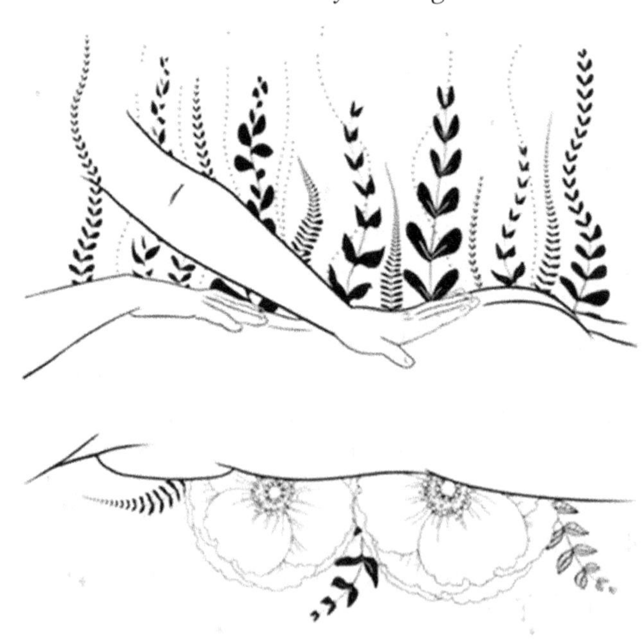

*Whole body massage.*

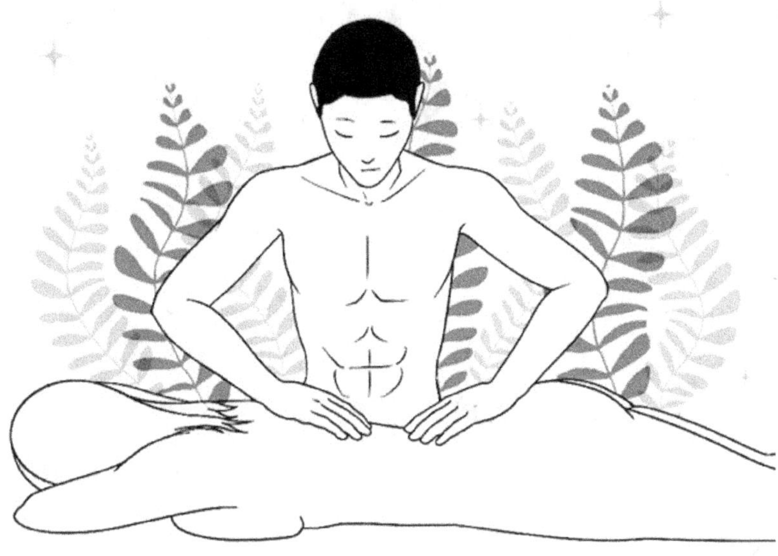

*Sexual energy merges with that of the heart.*

## Position 14

Caress her legs and massage her first chakra, freely moving your hands and caressing her with both your hands, alternating and using your fingertips to touch her. Then, slide your hands up to her head running all over her body. Work on the first Chakra, but also on the others.

Since an expert would be able to understand which spots need more attention than others, if you feel particularly interested in the topic, go on practicing it, to improve even more. This is just a taste and a mere explanation of the wide, deep purpose of tantra massage, and regardless of your level of awareness, the massage I am illustrating will be pleasant, complete, and exhaustive all the same if you stick to all the steps and do it with love and dedication. She will thank you for making her happy, and **you will be able to bring her to the ecstasy state of pleasure that she deserves.**

Now, it's time to turn her into a supine position, approaching her ear and whispering to her that it's time to turn around.

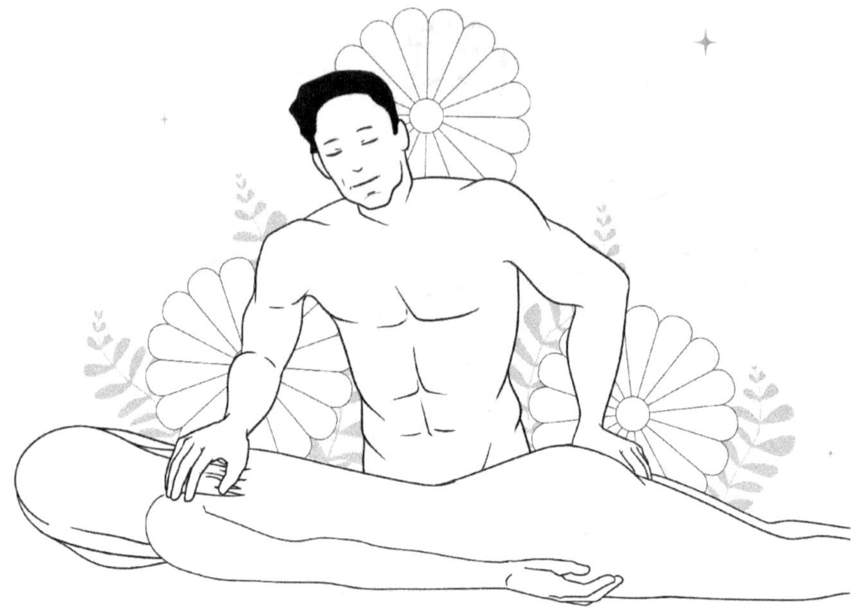

*Caress her Yoni and push the energy upwards, aws you massage the upper chakras with your other hand.*

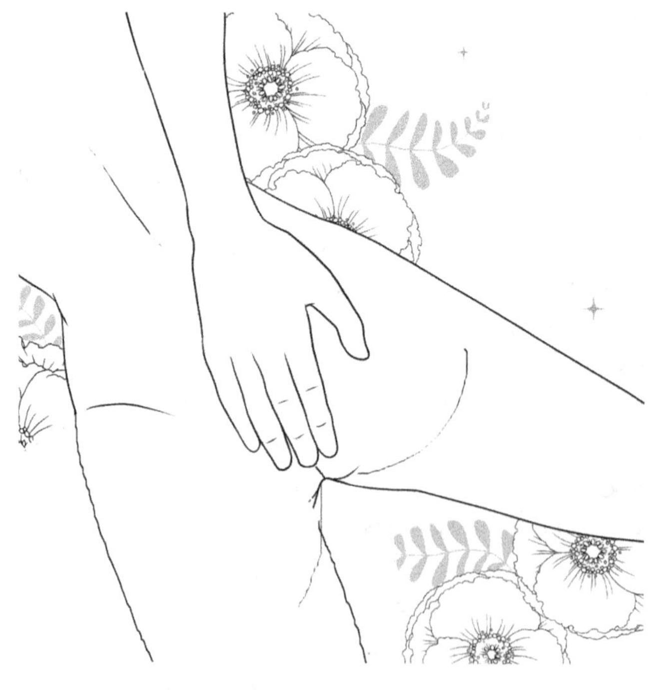

## 4 TIME: Position 15

Put your hand on the heart chakra and turn towards her, behind her head. Caress her using the scarf and let it slide over her body, bottom-top, playing a little. Then, stroke her all over the body, as far as you can go, while going up with your hands. Stroke her breast making circular movements around the nipple, getting in touch with her heart (below, an entire section dedicated to breast massage). Then, go from the heart to the throat, the communication chakra.

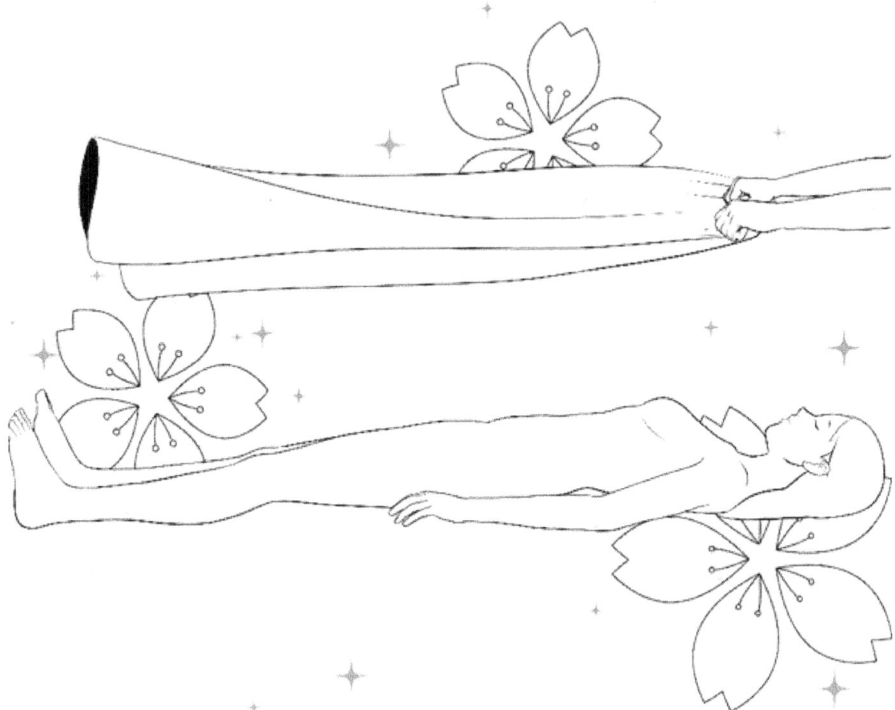

*Foulard massage.*

# Breast Massage as a Gate to the Heart and the Pineal Gland

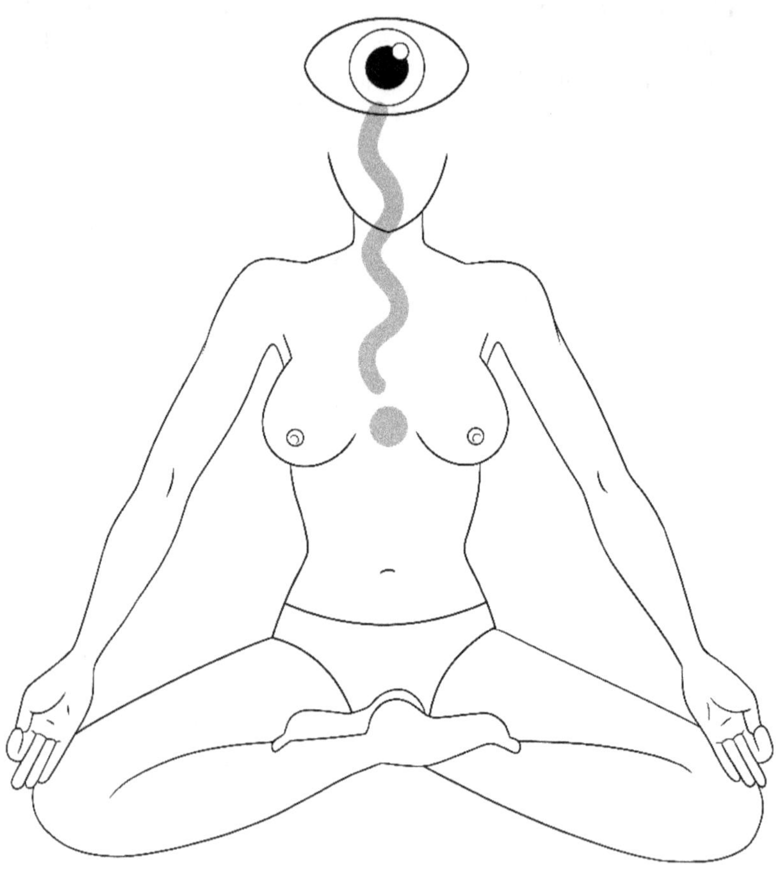

In the vast realm of Tantra Massage, an ancient and profound art that celebrates the body as a temple of energy and spiritual connection, a woman's breasts hold a sacred and powerful role. While the genitals are turned inward, the breast is the point of contact with the outside, the bridge between the earthly physicality and the deeper dimension of the heart and soul.

Through her breast, a woman can open her heart and connect with her emotional world, becoming able to control her emotions and giving her partner the possibility to get in touch with her most intimate feelings, for an authentic and deep kind of communication, supported by the energy of the heart.

In the sacred terminology of tantra, the breasts are also known as the "Snowy Mountains," "Peaches of Immortality," or "Corals," symbolizing fertility, beauty, and eternity.

When carrying out the massage, bring your hands to her breast to connect to her energy field and open yourself to love and union. Breathe, feel the sensations and impulses that the breast generates and the heartbeat that resonates through it.

Gently stroke her nipples, making circular movements outward, feeling the pineal gland awaken and opening the doors of perception and connection with the universe.

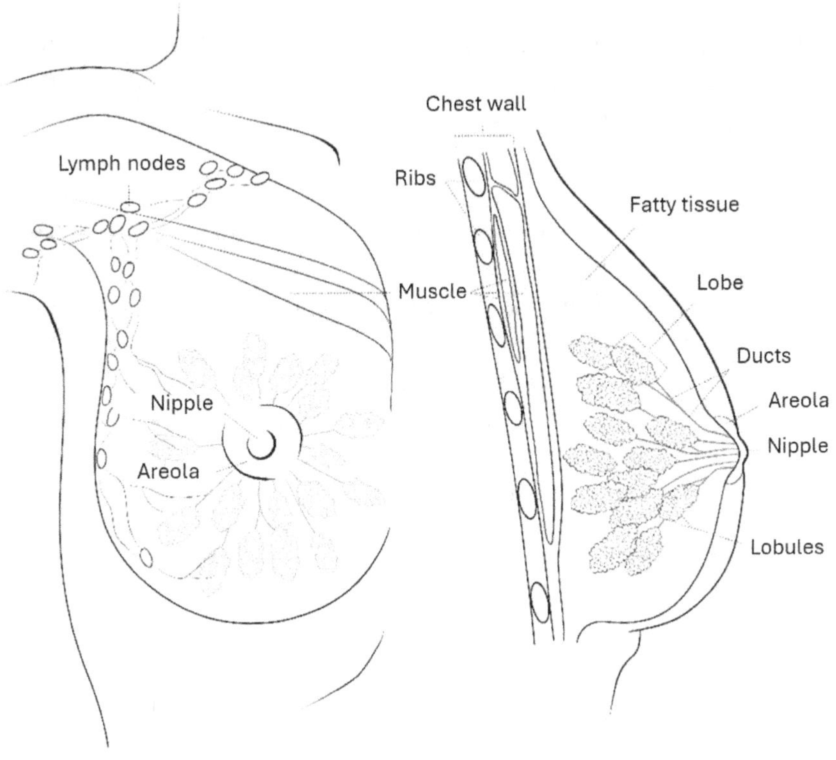

To massage the breasts and activate the pineal gland, you can try different types of touches:

## Breast Massage 1

1. Gently pour the oil on her breast, avoiding the nipples.
2. Put it on them with your hands.
3. Make wide movements, massaging the pectoral tissue with circular and wide movements, also including the shoulders and armpits, with constant contact.
4. Alternate small, circular movements with your fingers around the nipples first, and then moving closer and closer to involve them in the touch.

## Breast Massage 2

1. Hold the breast with one hand and gently squeeze it, but firmly.
2. Get lost in different types of caresses and pressures as you learn to listen to her body.
3. When touching the nipples, explore different kinds of stroking by rubbing, shaking, and holding them firmly between your fingers, while gradually increasing the pressure until you feel like you can stop.

## Breast Massage 3

1. Firmly grasp the nipples and let them vibrate with pressure, without releasing the nipple.
2. Repeat and let your whole hand vibrate, pinching it over and over again, then release.
3. Push the chest inward and massage it.
4. You can also use semi-melted ice cubes to further stimulate the sensitivity.
5. Try to alternate between these types of touches or focus on those that most resonate with the receiver, with respect, awareness, and love.

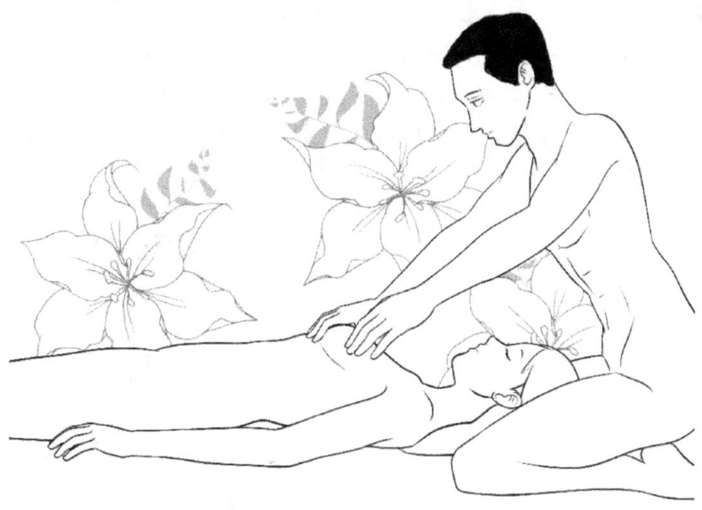

*Breast massage.*

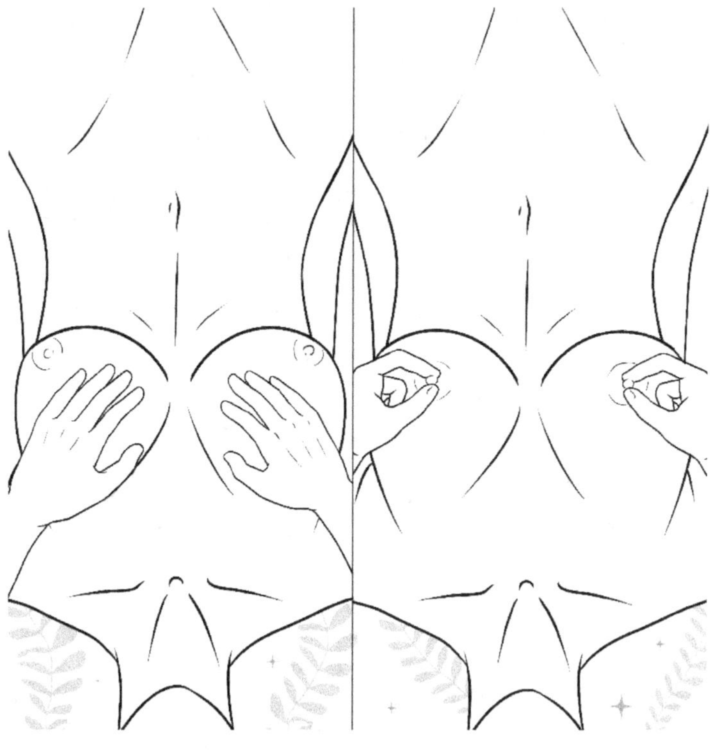

## Position 16

After massaging her, keep your hands open with your thumbs together on the third eye and breathe in sync with her. Remain like this for a few seconds, feel the powerful connection between you two, then switch your position and move to her right side.

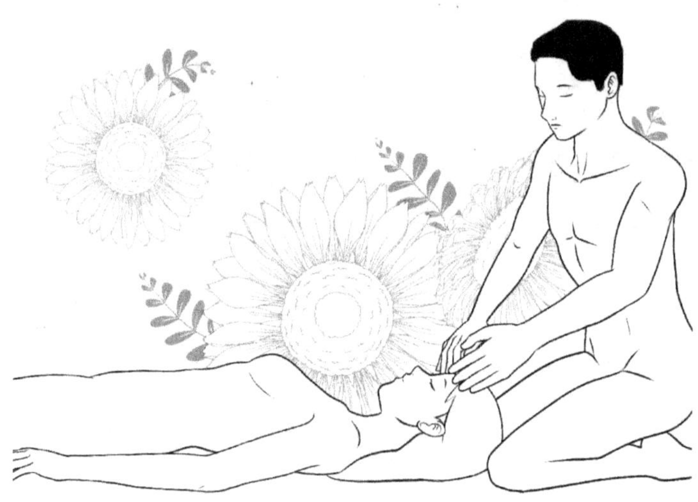

*Third eye massage, the pineal gland.*

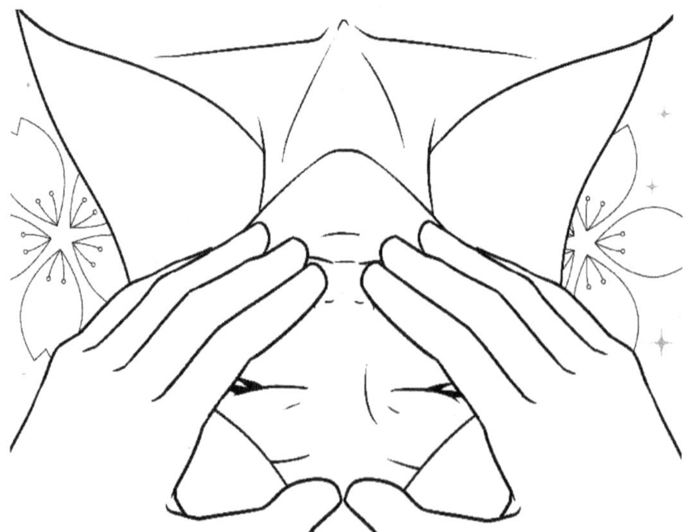

*Hands on the third eye, face, and crown.*

## 5 TIME: Position 17

Put your hand on her chest to keep the contact and turn towards her right side, then switch your position and caress her whole body, as you do every time, as shown in *Image A*.

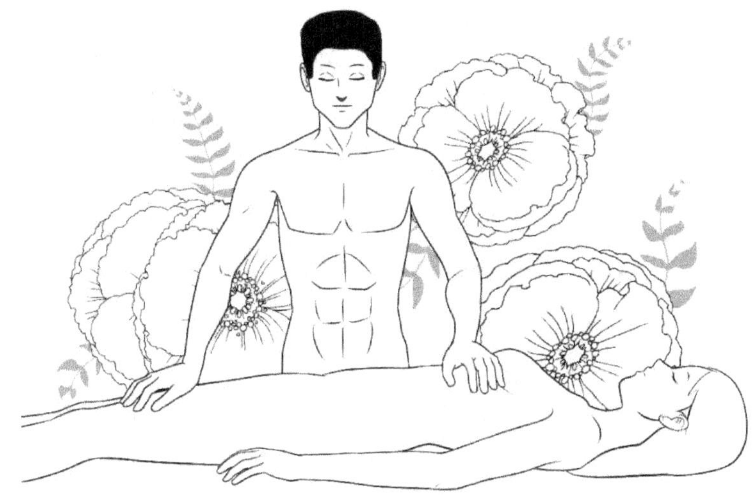

*5 TIME.*

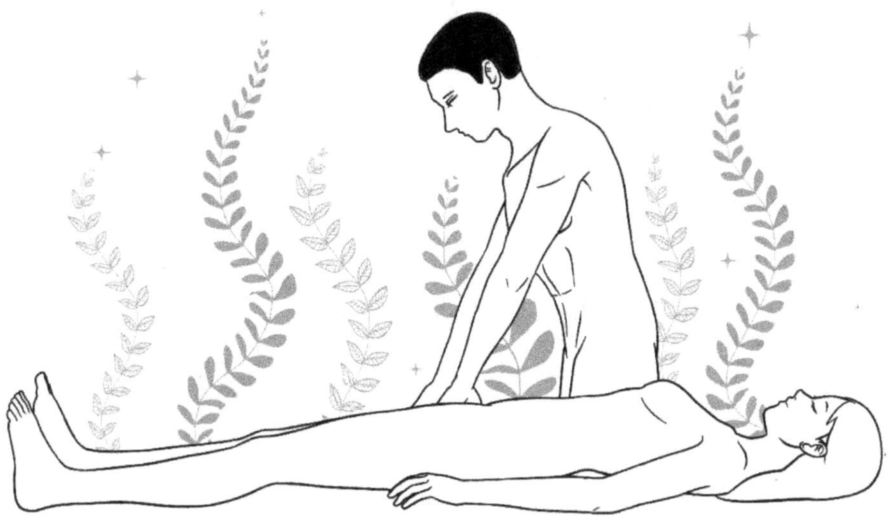

*Inner thigh massage and touch of Yoni.*

## Position 18

After massaging her whole body, touch and stimulate her first chakra but do not enter into her yet, until releasing all her sexual energy. Caress her labia majora and play with your fingertips, while feeling the breath and pleasure that gets released, as well as the awakening of her sexual energy. After that, gently spread her legs and enter with yours. You can choose between the two positions shown below, according to what is most comfortable for you. Do you prefer to be on your knees or with your legs crossed to hers? Either way, once positioned start massaging her legs, from her feet to her vulva

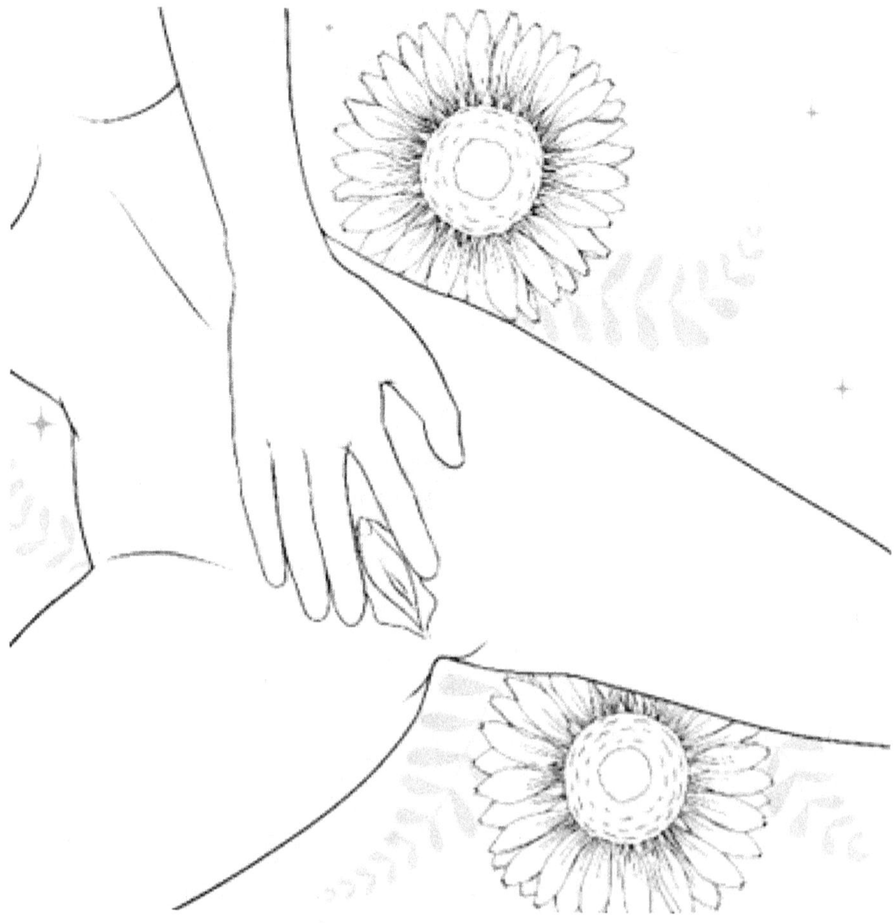

*Light caresses of the external parts of the Yoni.*

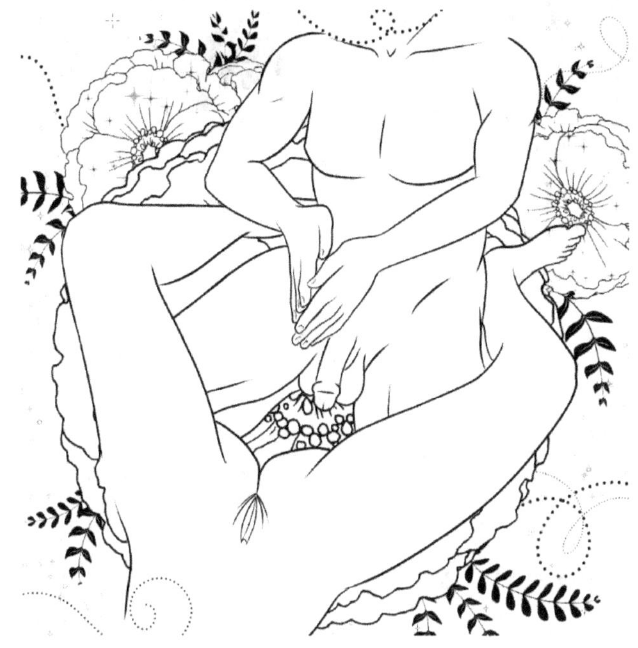

*1. Enter inside her legs, from here start focusing on her Yoni*

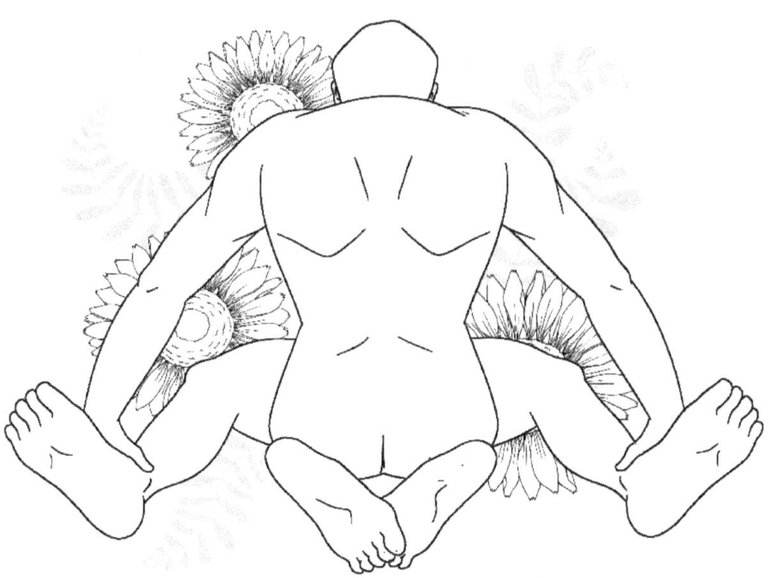

*Leg massage from feet to Yoni.*

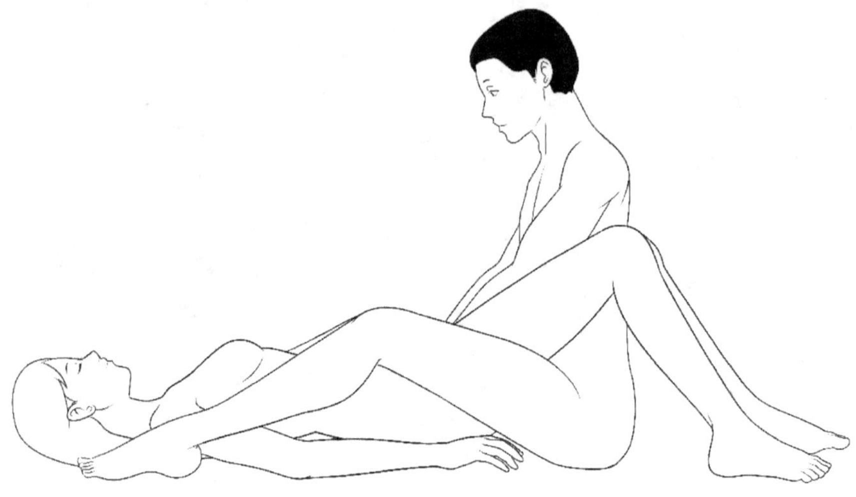

*2. Enter her legs, starting to fully focus on her Yoni.*

# 5. Discovering Yoni's Sacred Anatomy

## *Explore the Vulvar's Most Sensible Zones*

**B**efore starting to talk about Yoni massage, you should know a bit more about the different erogenous zones we will be referring to in this guide and the types of orgasms women can experience.

Below, the anatomy of the female genitals

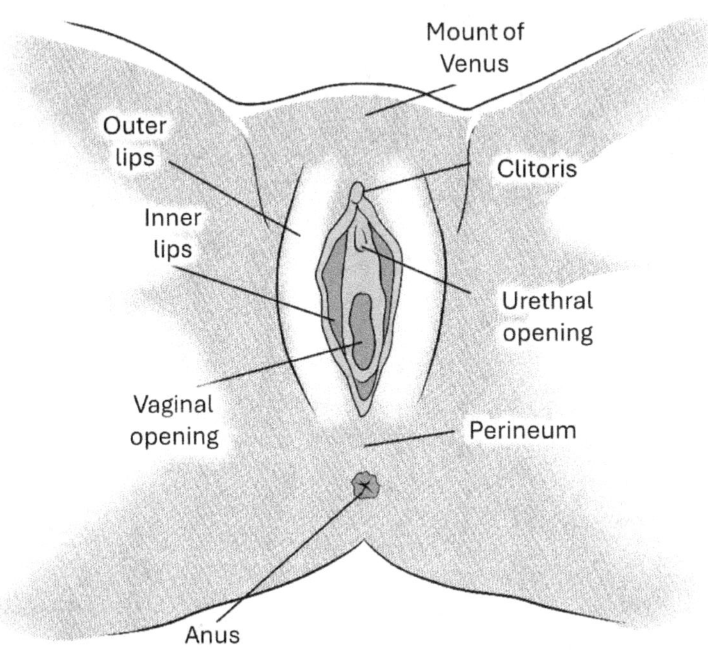

Like our feet, hands and other parts of the body, the Yoni also has its reflex zones connected to certain internal organs. *Reflexology* has its roots in traditional Chinese medicine, as we have anticipated, and consists of the targeted stimulation of certain reflex points of the body that are crossed by what are called energy meridians connected to the internal organs. In practice, the stimulation of the Yoni will bring well-being to the whole body, even on an emotional level, and not just to the treated area.

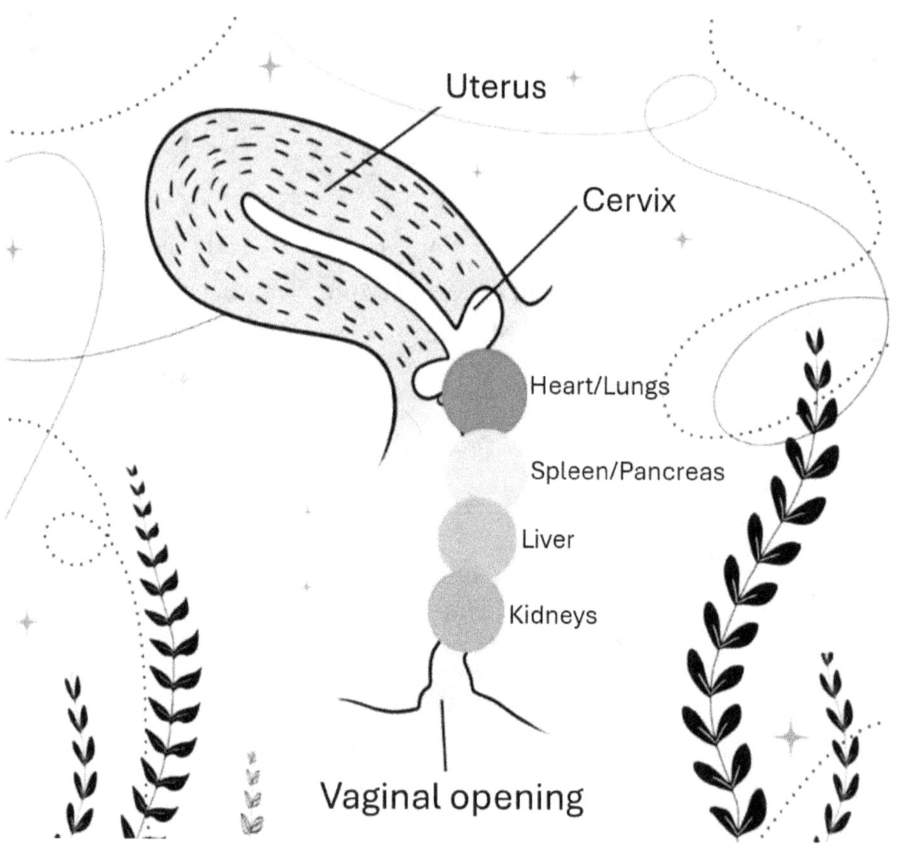

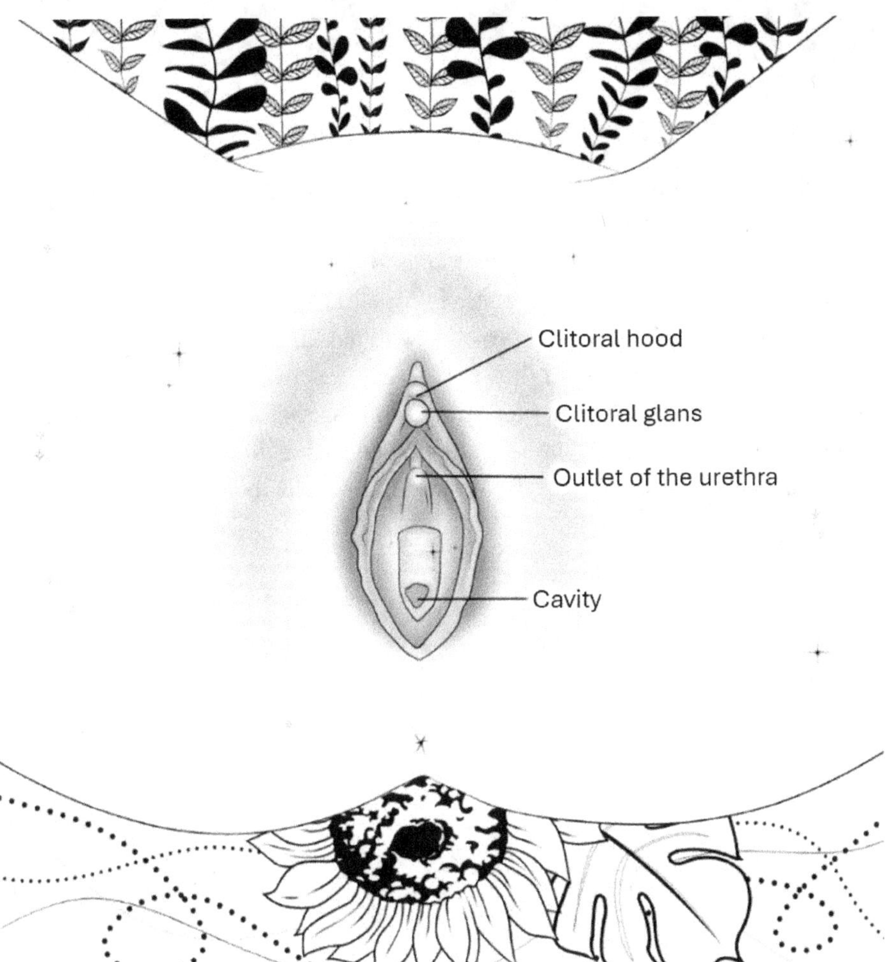


In proximity to the region of Lingam, the male sexual organ, there are some reflex zones too. During sex, these zones get activated, creating a mutual stimulation that spreads throughout the whole body, for a feeling of diffused pleasure and contributing to a general sense of well-being and harmony. Through the Yoni massage, these areas get treated in a deep way to release physical and emotional tensions, thus leading to natural relaxation and increased vitality. Over time, this treatment can also improve our ability to experience pleasure and develop a greater orgasmic potential.

The inner lips are formed by internal folds and gather in a kind of hood containing the clitoris pearl, the outer part of it, and the glans, and it is possible to easily touch it since it is located just above the inner lips.

# Female Orgasm: How Many Types Are There?

Orgasm moment is unique and extraordinary; when all of the emotions and physical sensations get so merged and combined that it is difficult to describe with words. When women experience orgasm, their emotions get transformed and their body undergoes surprising changes at a physiological level. Yoni opens and expands, while the erectile tissue of the clitoris fills with blood, greatly increasing the size of the clitoral pearl. Along with this, the uterus rises towards the abdomen, while the nipples become erect and darker. All these physical changes are surprising and unique phenomena, which emphasize the wonder and complexity of the female body. During this process, the sexual tension gradually increases, pervading the

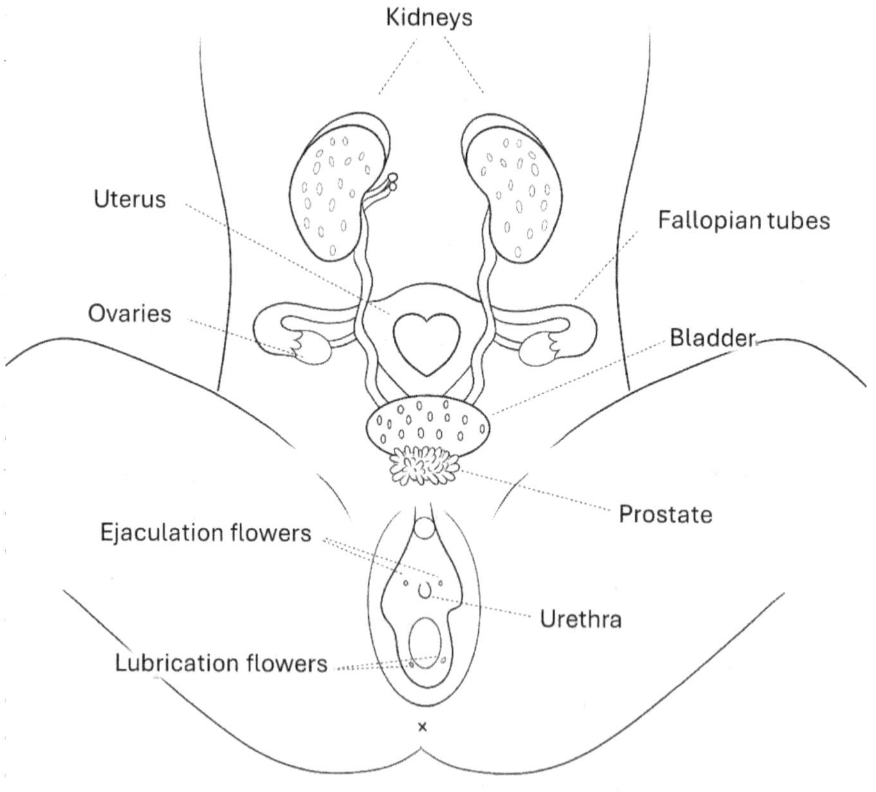

# Discovering Amrita: The Sacred Fluid of Female Ejaculation

Before we get into the wonderful world of Yoni massage, it is good for us to tackle the concept of female ejaculation, known as "Sacred Water" in sacred sexuality terms.

In the wide universe of sacred sexuality, there is an ancient and precious mystery present in the tradition of *Amrita*, the female ejaculation liquid. Also known as the nectar of the gods, it is more than just a bodily fluid since it is a symbol of transformation and spiritual connection that goes beyond mere cultures or centuries. Sacred sexuality is a thousand-year journey that unites the spiritual and the flesh, rooted in the ancient tantric practices of India and the sacred rites of ancient Egypt, as well as in the traditions of ancient Greece and Rome.

This concept has been evolving over the centuries, influencing cultures and traditions all over the world. In the 20th century, it experienced a significant renaissance through the movement of New Thought and sexual awareness, leading to a growing interest in the exploration of the connection between sexuality and spirituality. It is much more than a mere physical act; it is a true awakening of the creative sexual energy that leads to a unified kind of awareness. Through the body, mind, and heart, we can learn to transform this energy into a spiritual and creative experience that permeates every area of our lives!

## An Invitation to Awareness: Sacred Sexuality as a Spiritual Path

Opening to the potential of sacred sexuality means embracing sex as a spiritual and consciousness-expanding path. It is making love to yourself and the entire universe, integrating your mind, heart, and sex into one creative intention.

In this quest for sexual and spiritual awareness, we encounter Amrita, the sacred fluid of female ejaculation, which represents the quintessence of sacred sexuality and its connection to the divine.

In a realm where sensuality is sacred and female pleasure is celebrated as a divine manifestation, there is an ancient and precious mystery: Amrita. This fluid, which flows from the very source of female pleasure, is more than just a bodily fluid. It is an act of devotion to the inner divinity that resides within every woman, a sacred connection that extends far beyond the confines of the physical body.

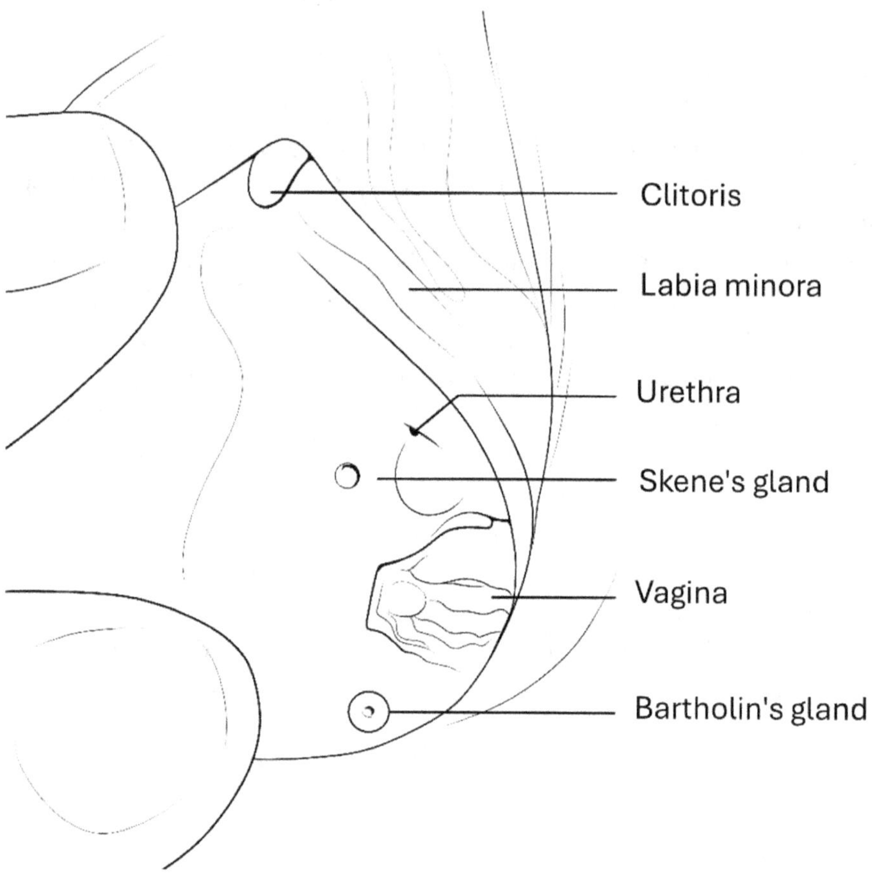


*Inner parts of the vagina.*

## Four Main Fluids Concerning Women

- Vaginal lubricant, before and during orgasm.
- Lubricant glands, during orgasm.
- Female ejaculation occurs in the woman's prostate.
- Oral ejaculation.

Female ejaculation is related to the paraurethral glands. The orgasm that is reached when the woman ejaculates causes an involuntary segregation of abundant liquid, which forms in the female prostate. Its texture, smell, and taste are different from urine since it is a tasteless, colorless liquid with no smell.

Female ejaculation is expelled during sexual intercourse or in moments of high pleasure, even though never before the beginning of the act itself, as in the case of natural lubricating liquid. Indeed, it is absolutely normal for a woman to feel the need to urinate when she is about to ejaculate or when the prostate is stimulated, even though the valve that opens and closes the connection between the bladder and urethra closes, making her unable to urinate. Vulvas that do not manifest visible ejaculations are ejaculating inward, and the liquid ends up in the bladder, being urinated immediately after orgasm or stimulation.

*Amrita* is a true ritual of divine connection, a balm that gives immortality to those who drink from it. Through it, women share their divinity state with themselves and their partners, creating a spiritual connection that goes beyond the boundaries of the flesh. The sacred waters of the *Amrita* not only contain pleasure but also vital energy and hormones that are the key to eternal youth and longevity.

## The Female Prostate as the Sacred Pont

This point is located on the vagina, just below the bladder (see pictures above). The prostate is connected to two holes, one on each side of the urethra, through which women ejaculate. Since the bladder connects to the urethra, it is not pee, and the sensations experienced in this part are connected to the pelvic floor, located above the vagina. To stimulate it, all you have to do is enter with your fingers (index and middle) into the vagina, when she is aroused, and press towards the pubic bone.

## The Awakening of Kundalini Energy: The Amrita Way

The mystery of *Amrita* is linked to kundalini energy, the sacred snake residing at the base of the spine. Through the massage of the "sacred point" or female prostate (also called G-spot), women can awaken this powerful energy, guiding it along the central axis of their being. Through gentle and conscious movements, they can bring *Amrita* out of its source to its apex, nourishing all the other energy centers along the way. This is not just a moment of ecstatic pleasure, but also an act of self-expression and freedom. Through the "sacred point" massage, women can learn to connect more deeply with their body and sexuality, overcoming mental blocks and prejudices that might hinder their enjoyment; with regular practice and a higher level of body awareness, every woman can reach her *Amrita* and experience its transformative power!

## Amrita Buccal Journey: The Awakening of the Divine Taste Buds

As we said, *Amrita* is not only a physical experience but also a sensory and spiritual one. By practicing *kechari mudra*, women can awaken their divine taste buds and savor the nectar of eternity. Through gentle and conscious movements of the tongue, they can activate their palate and enjoy the pleasure of *Amrita* buccal. With confidence and love for themselves, every woman can start this journey to immortality and ecstatic bliss.

# 6. Yoni Massage, Awaken Your Sexual Energy

## Step-by-Step Yoni Massage

After gently massaging her whole body and going around her, return between her legs. Spread her thighs and place yours between them, making sure they are slightly bent and spread to properly expose the Yoni area.

From this position, the real Yoni massage begins. You can keep your partner's legs fully extended to help her relax or kneel if it feels more comfortable. It is important to proceed only when the woman is completely relaxed and aroused, to tackle the vulva area and make sure there is a good atmosphere to start.

During this phase, the main goal is to awaken the female sexual energy by creating a wave of pleasure, an ecstatic **dance permeating her whole body, preparing it for the following phases, that will concentrate on Yoni.**

# External Vulvar Massage: Be Open-Minded, Active, and Full of Energies

## Preparation

The masseur stands at the woman's feet, in one of the two positions seen at the end of the previous chapter, and places his hands on her ankles. Bring his hands to the woman's hips with his thumbs between her legs, passing through the Yoni. (Go up and down 3 times). The reclining recipient gently rests the woman's legs on his outstretched legs, allowing her to let them fall comfortably. Place his hands in Namaste' in reverence to the Yoni, then rest them on her. First the left hand, then the right hand.

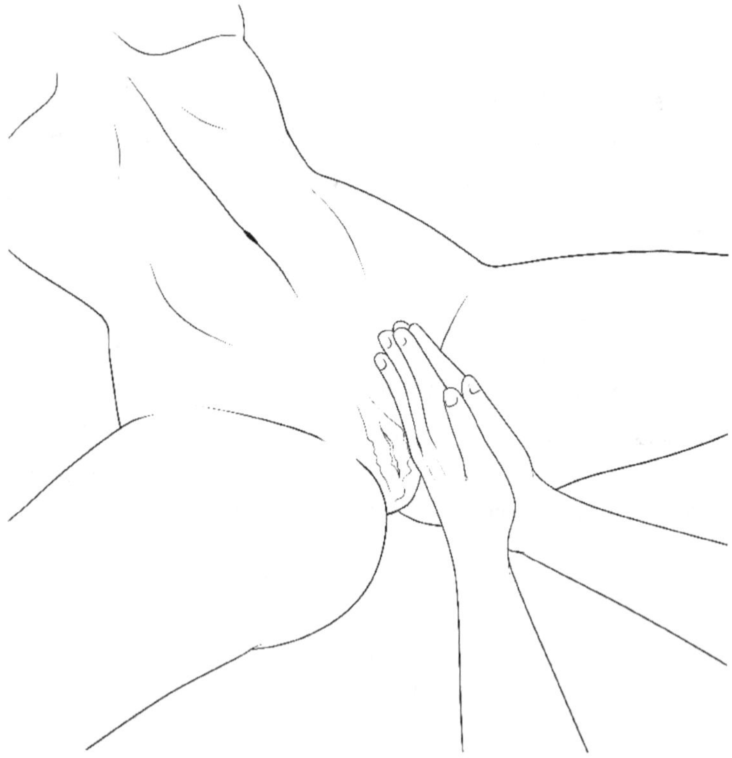

*Hands in Namaste' in reverence towards the Yoni.*

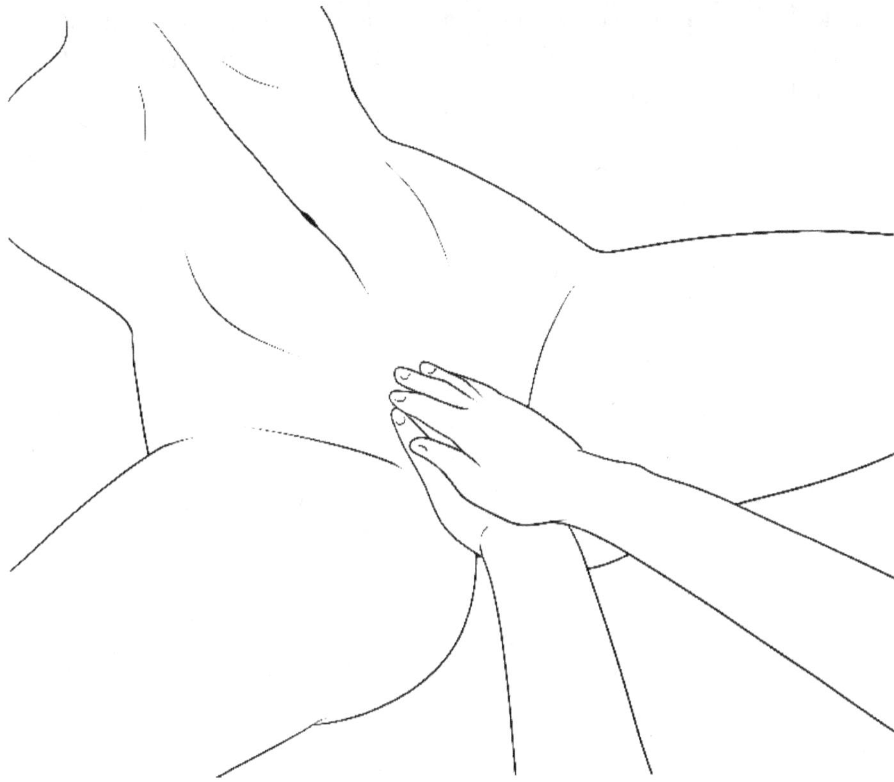

*Hands placed on her, first the left hand, then the right hand.*

## The Venus Spin

In the Tantric Massage, with the Venus Spin expression, we tend to refer to a series of gentle and loving techniques aimed at awakening and harmonizing the female energy. By following these simple steps, you can create a relaxing and deeply connected experience for your partner. Here's how to perform it:

- **Oil**—Pour some oil on her mount of Venus and make three circles, then gently pour more on Yoni until it is completely covered.
- **Heaven-earth connection**—Pour some oil on her stomach and make three circles, then go gently down towards the mount of Venus, first with one hand and then with the other, and do the same in the opposite direction; then, starting from Yoni towards the stomach. This way, you will be connecting earth to heaven!

- **Clock**—Place the heel of your left hand on the pubic clockwise, at 12 o'clock, and drag it to the tip of your fingers. Then, at 3 o'clock, and drag it. Finally, at 9 o'clock, and drag it.

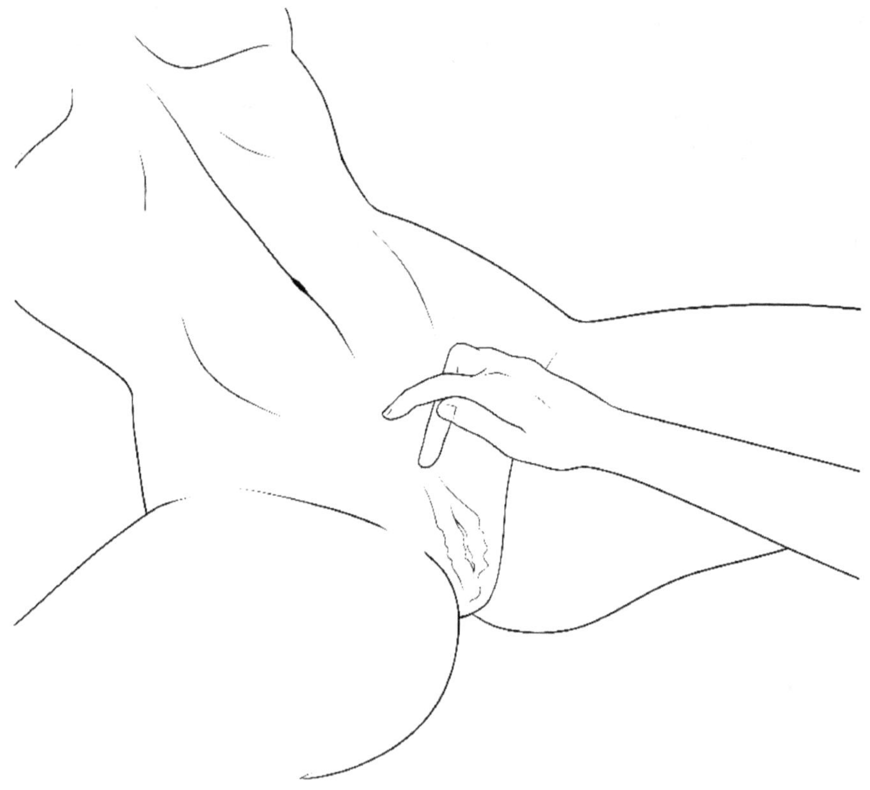

*Pour some oil on the mount of Venus.*

- **Clock**—Place the heel of your left hand on the pubic clockwise, at 12 o'clock, and drag it to the tip of your fingers. Then, at 3 o'clock, and drag it. Finally, at 9 o'clock, and drag it.

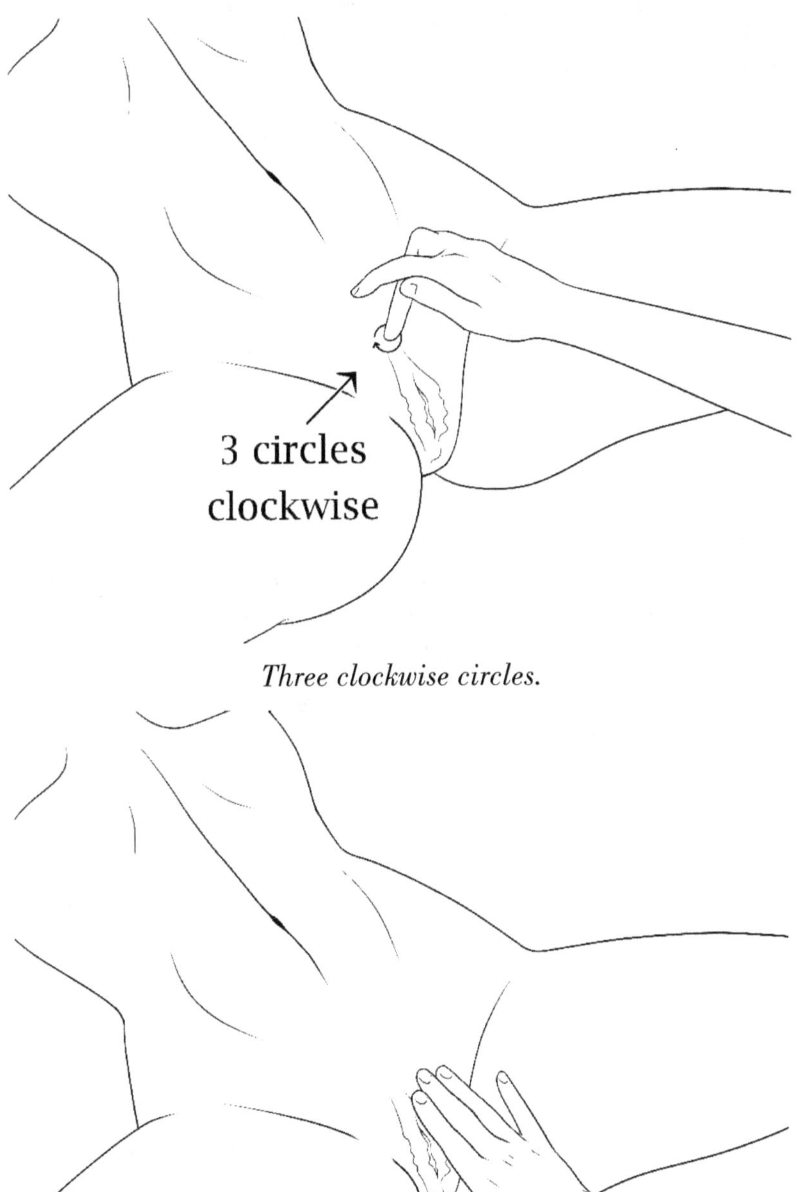



*Three clockwise circles.*

*Cover the Yoni with the oil and pat gently.*

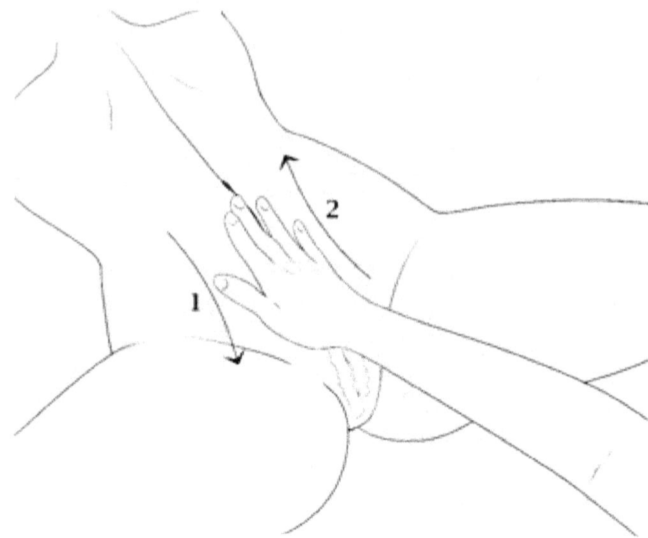

*Gentle massage from the stomach, 12 o'clock direction, towards the mount of Venus and vice versa, first with one hand and then with the other.*

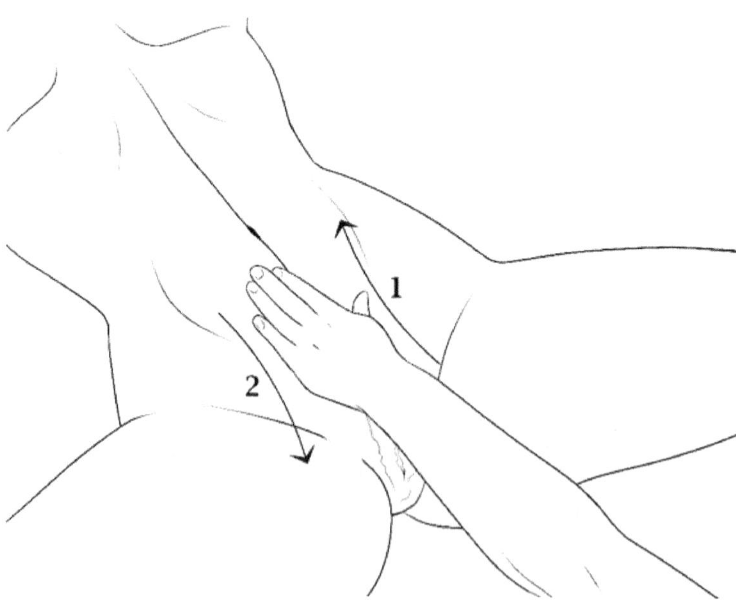

*Gentle massage from Yoni to the stomach and vice versa, first with one hand and then with the other.*

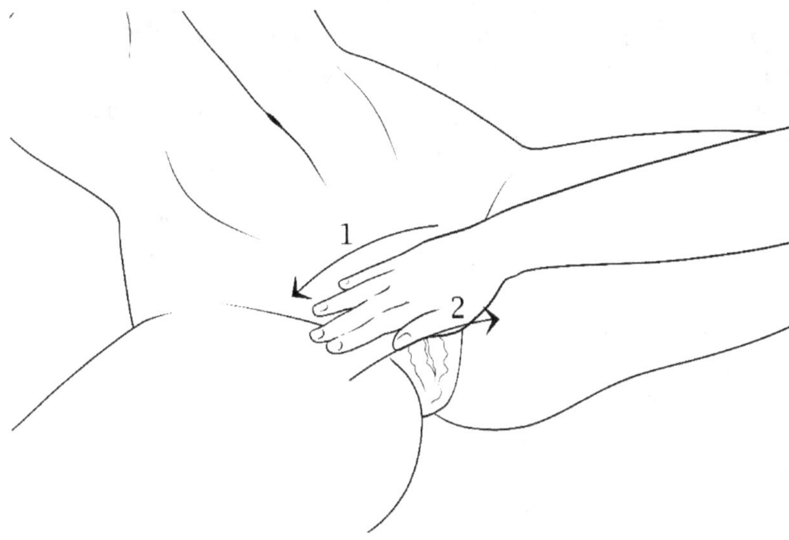

*Yoni gentle massage, from 3 o'clock direction to 9 o'clock and vice versa, first with one hand and then with the other.*

## Yoni External Massage

Before fully entering Yoni, it is important to perform an external massage to make the receiver and her first Chakra familiar with our presence. Starting from the mount of Venus and going towards the stomach, the aim is to open Yoni, activate it, and awaken it by giving energy to it. Now, imagine dividing the vulva into six zones, six half-moons; each zone will be treated with:

- Three very slow opening strokes followed by three faster closing strokes (open).
- Three movements in very slow circles followed by three faster closing strokes (activate).
- Three very slow pressure movements followed by three faster closing strokes (energy).

Remember that the opening movements should be synchronized with your exhalation and the closing ones with your inspiration, as well as your breathing, which should follow that of the receiver.

The six half-moons representing the six areas to be treated are illustrated below. The chronological direction indicated by the numbers and the path to be followed by the hands indicated by the opening and closing signs indicate which movement to do first (for example, movement 1 goes from left to right, and closes from right to left, as indicated below, and so on for other areas). Each area should be treated first with a caress three times **(open)**, then with circular movements **(activate)**, and finally with pressures **(feel-wake)**. Do not forget about the natural oil while doing all this. Below, you will find the image and then the right process to treat a specific area, which will be the same for all the others. After each explanation, images will help you understand the movements, positions, and touches.

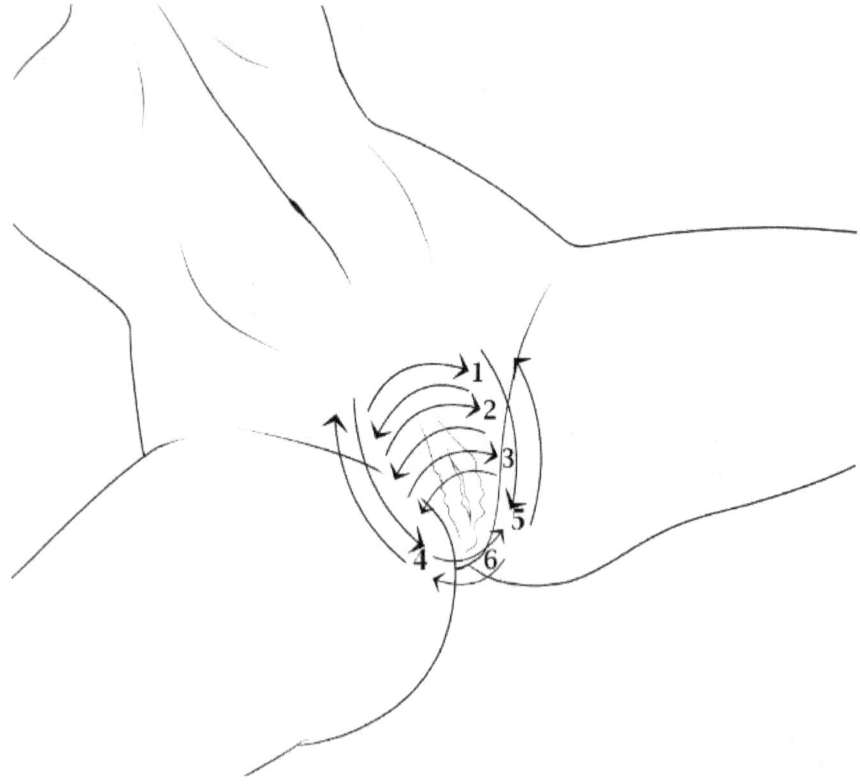

**Area 1:** It represents the first half-moon, the mount of Venus. **Open** it with a stroke from left to right as you exhale, using one or two fingers and returning to the starting point with an open-hand stroke as you inhale. Use the hand that you prefer, remembering that the opening stroke must preferably be performed with the tip of a finger, or two, whilst the closing one is with the open hand and with all fingers. Always remember to follow the partner's breath and to perform the movement three times, always trying to look into your partner's eyes even if she closes them.

Now, remaining in the same area, **activate** Yoni following the same procedure, but just using one or two fingers, with small, clockwise circles, and very gently and slowly. Follow the path of the half moon, from left to right, and then close with a stroke from right to left in a more determined way, remembering that your breathing must always be synchronized with that of the receiver. Perform this three times, looking into the other's eyes.

Remain in that half-moon area and give Yoni new energies through pressures, pressing with a finger while following the same path, then releasing it a quarter inch away from one point to the next, softly and always from left to right. Next, come back with a hand stroke firmly open. Perform this movement three times.

Now that you have completed the first half-moon, perform the same procedure in zone one, three, four, and so on until the sixth, which is the perineum area, i.e., between the vagina and anus. Do not be in a hurry to enter, but remember that the vulva also has many external receptors; awakening these points could be the key to a new kind of relaxation and pleasure never experienced before! If certain areas of your partner hurt during the pressures, they may be the ones that need the most attention. Invite the receiver to release this pain during the open-mouth exhalation, emanating a liberation exclamation.

Below are some illustrations representing these three phases:

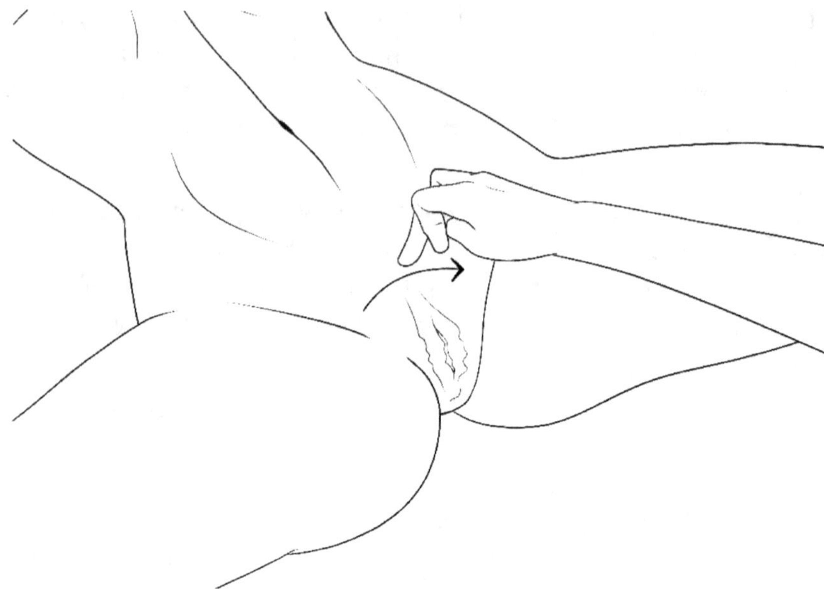

*Gentle opening caress with fingertips from left to right while exhaling.*

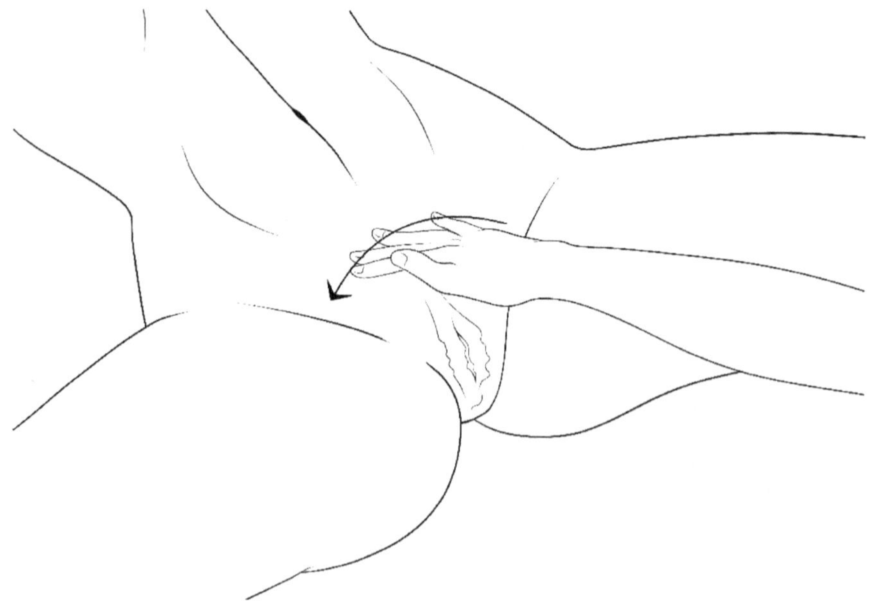

*Firm closing stroke from right to left, while inhaling.*

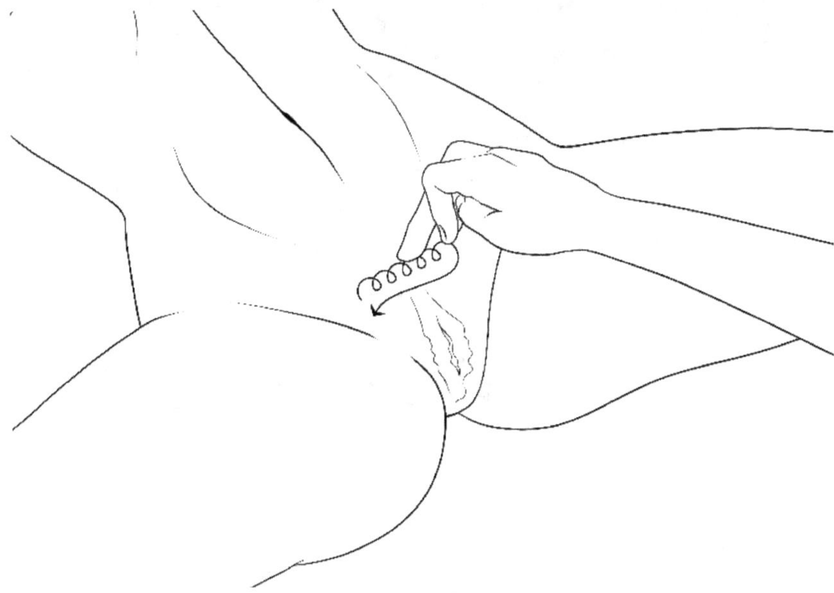

*Gently massage in circular movements from left to right, while exhaling.*

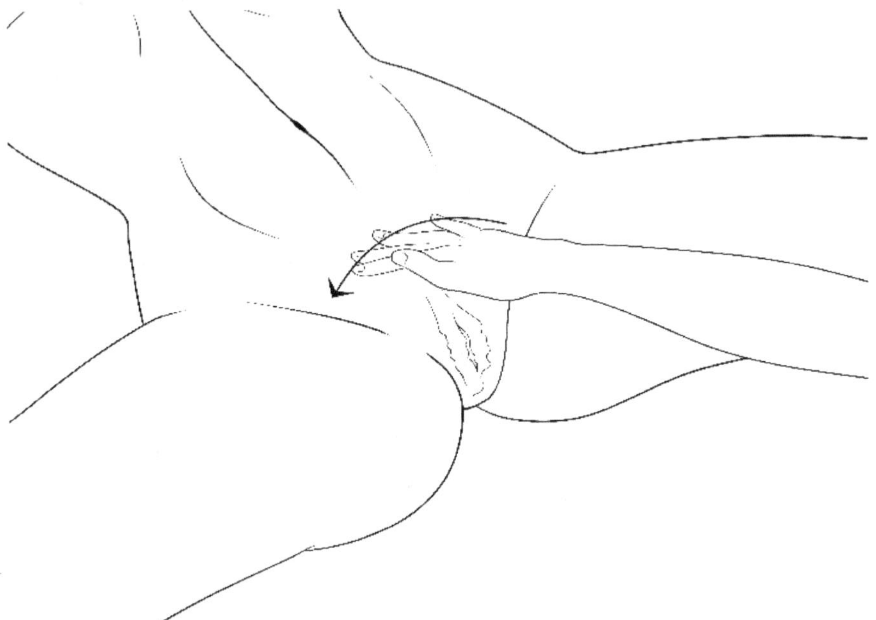

*Firm closing stroke from right to left, as you inhale.*

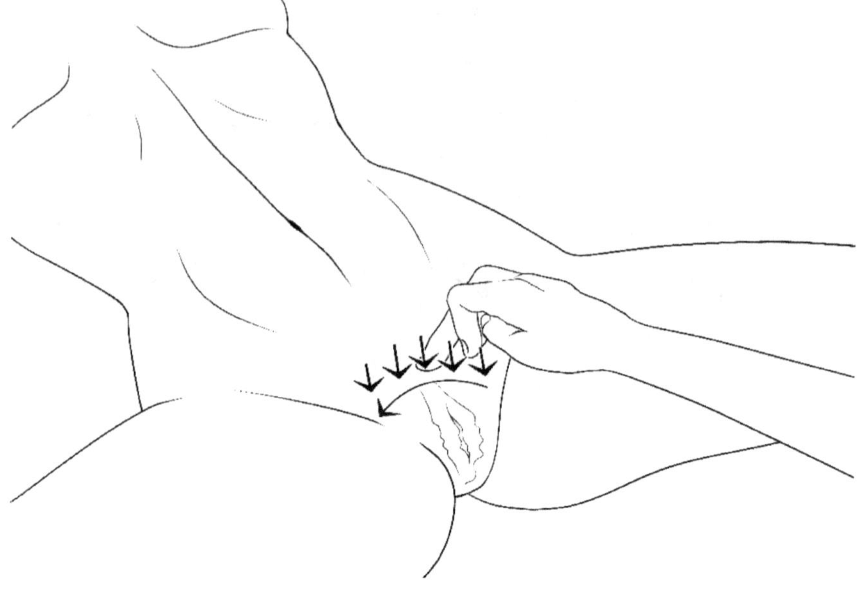

*Strengthening pressures from right to left.*

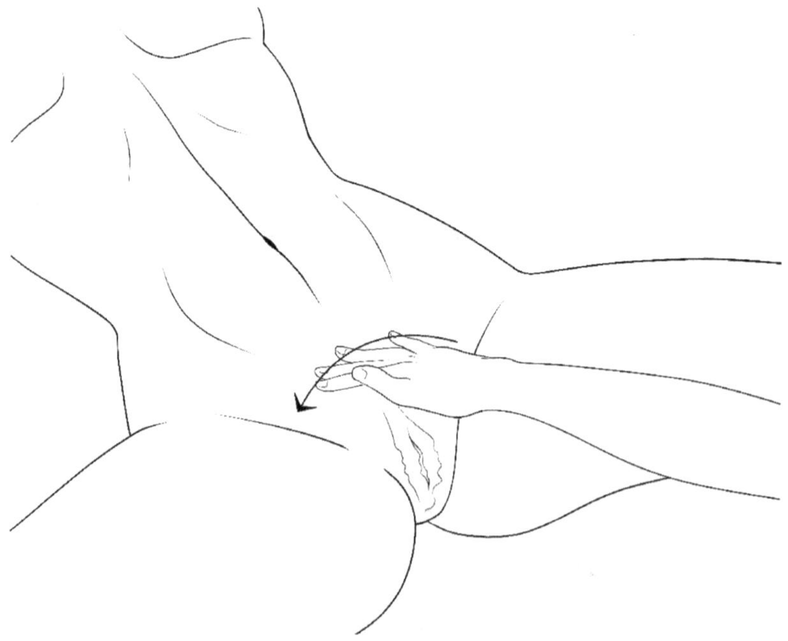

*Firm closing stroke from right to left.*

Now repeat these three steps three times on all six areas, half-moons, after which you can finally start to stimulate the Yoni with two-finger pressure in its central axis where the right and left lips meet. Start pressing from the bottom then in correspondence with the perineum up to the mons pubis in a slow and gentle manner always synchronizing your breathing and remember when you press exhale, when you release, inhale always synchronized with the breathing of the receiver.

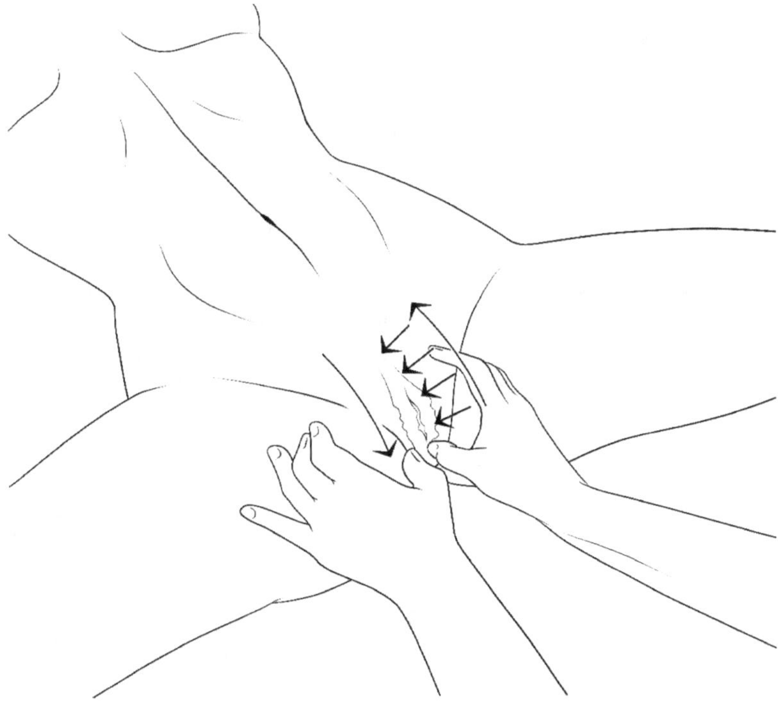

*Pressures on Yoni's central axis.*

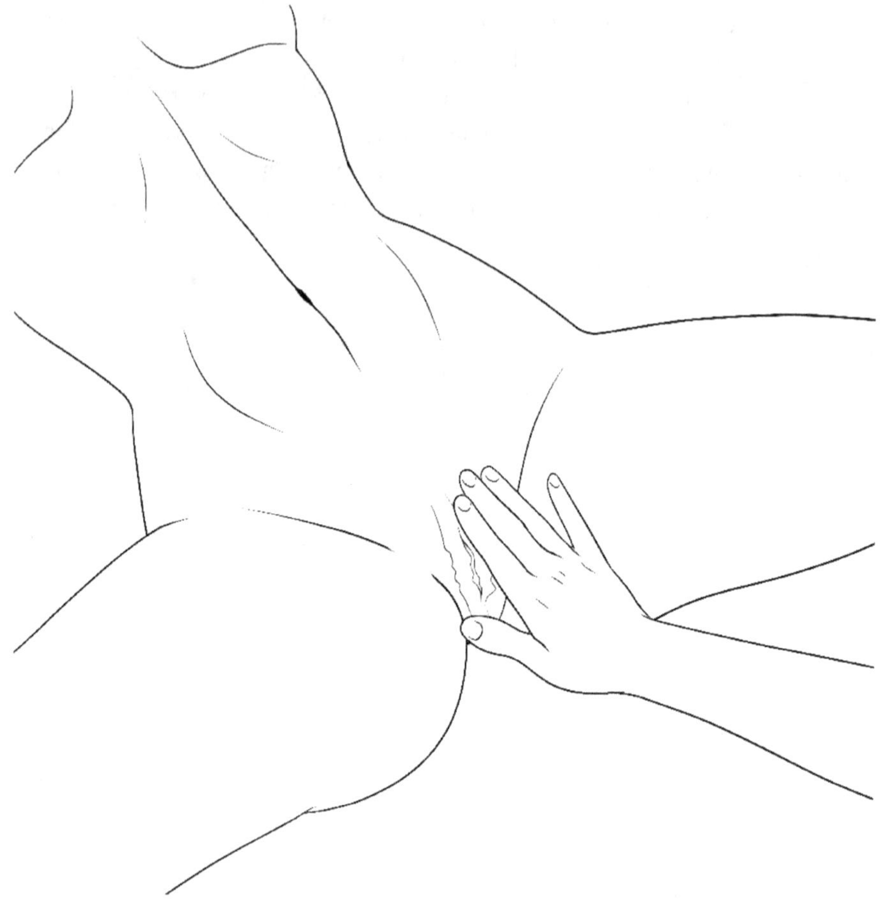

*Closing stroke from the top to the bottom.*

## Labia Majora and Minora Massage

Place your right hand on Yoni and your left one at the center of the receiver's chest, deeply breathing for at least a minute, to create an energetic connection between Yoni and the heart.

Slide your palms from her hips to the mount of Venus, until they are joined one by another, just above the pubis.

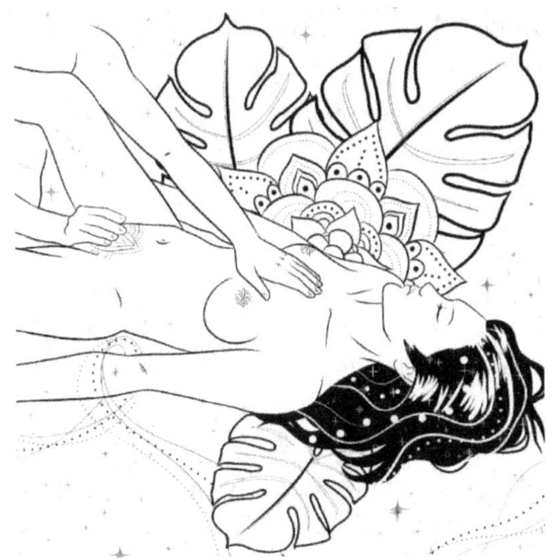

*Your right hand is on Yoni and your left one is at the center of her chest.*

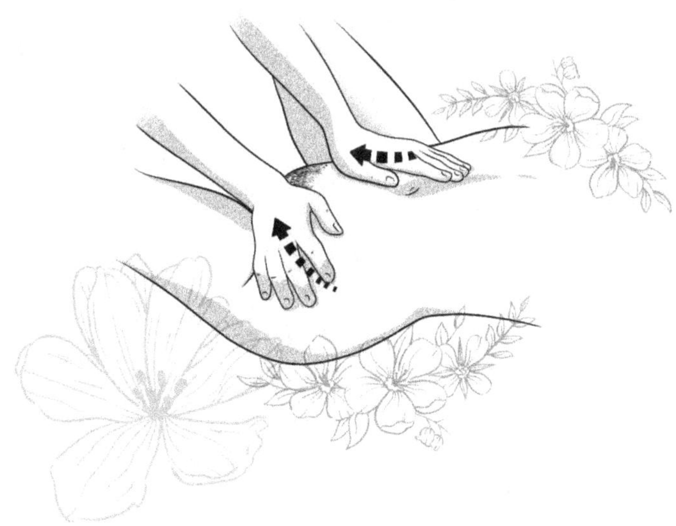

**Slide the palms from the stomach to the mons pubis...**

Now, it is time to open Yoni with sweetness, delicacy, and sensuality. In this second phase, the massage has to be carried out externally through the mount of Venus and the outer (labia majora) and inner lips (labia minora).

Pour some oil on your hands and start massaging the mount of Venus with circular movements and a light touch.

Using your fingertips, perform drum movements on the mount of Venus area and the surrounding area of the lower abdomen as if you were playing piano with quick and gentle touches.

Slide up and down the lips by moistening them with a light layer of oil.

Gently place the thumbs along the outer sides of the labia majora, starting at the base. The left thumb exerts light pressure on the left side, while the right thumb exerts light pressure on the right side. Applying a thin pressure, similar to a more intense stroke, simultaneously slide the thumbs up along the edge of the labia majora to their top. From there, gently rewind, following the path of the outer lips downwards to the base of the Yoni. Repeat this movement several times, alternating between up and down motion for a smooth and pleasant sensation.

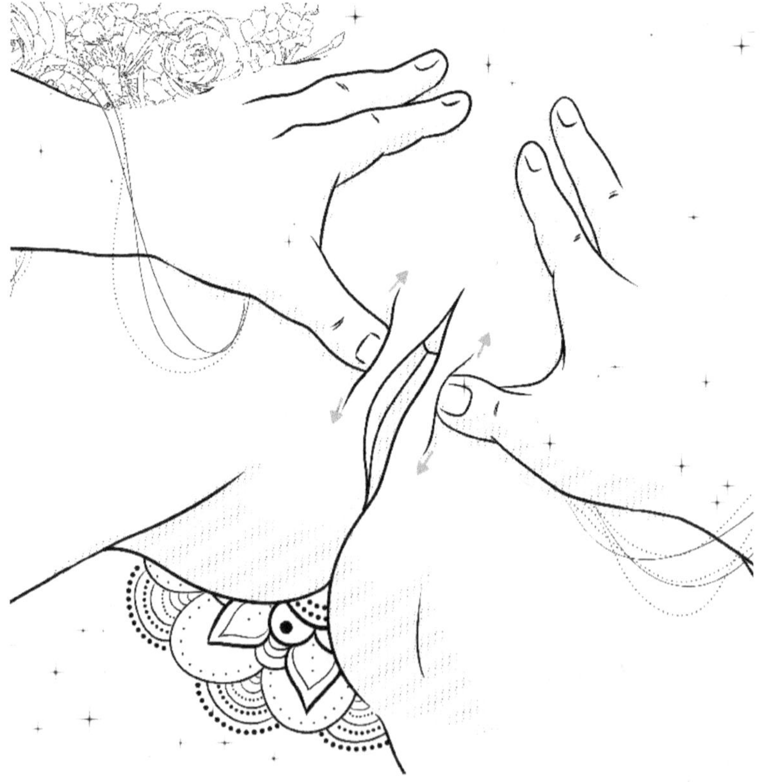

*Sliding the thumbs from top to bottom and vice versa along the labia majora.*

Delicately pinch and squeeze the labia majora using the index finger and thumb of the same hand, pressing it slightly, to stimulate by lifting the lip edge. Once it is pressed, release it and then gently pinch again with a continuous movement, over and over again.

Do the same for the entire lip edge, going up from bottom to top and then back down. Start on one side of the lips, right or left, then go to the other side. You can also treat the edges of the lips with both hands as in the picture.

The required time does not have to be fixed in advance, as it is important to follow the receiver's breath and connection, which allows you to understand whether to continue with the same technique or move on to the next step. Afterward, you will have to repeat the previous two steps on the labia minora, and then again on both labia majora and minora, at the same time.

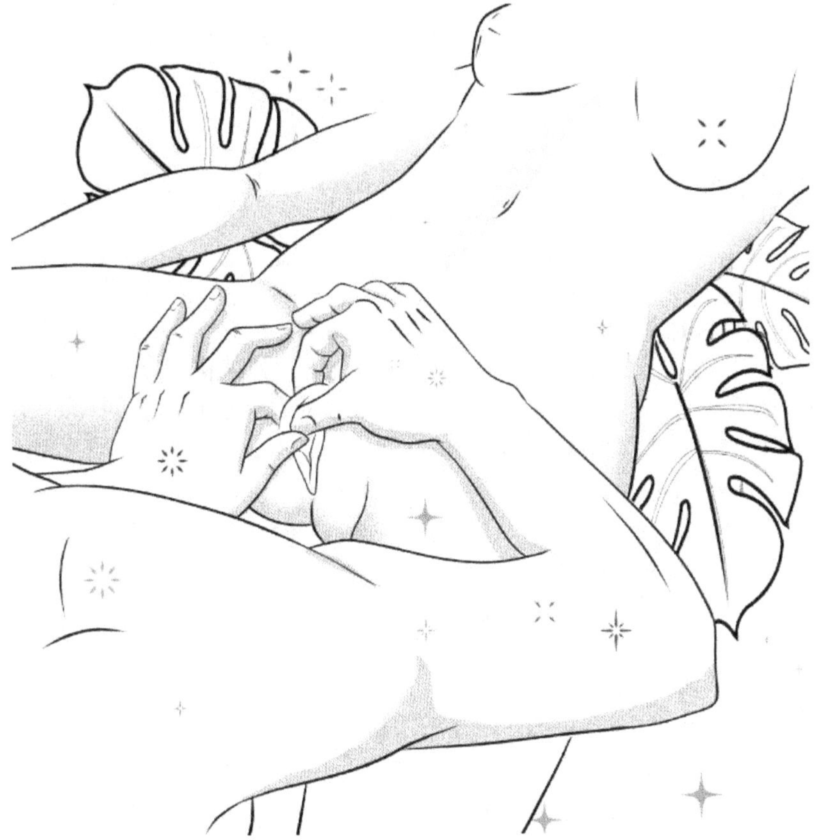

*Squeeze and pinch the labia majora and minora.*

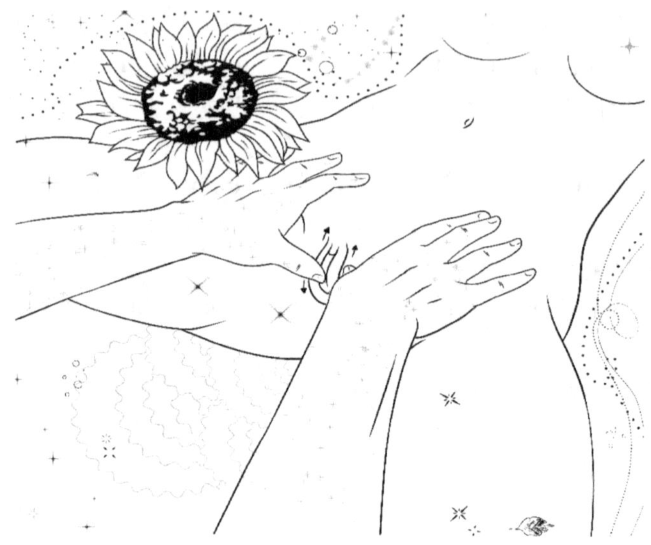

*Slipping of labia majora and minora.*

## Clitoral Massage

Now you can start massaging the clitoris, a highly sensitive organ located at the top of the Yoni, as illustrated above in the female anatomy. With nearly 8,000 nerve endings, the clitoris is one of the most complex organs in the female body, far exceeding the number found in the male glans penis by four times. These extremely delicate sensory nerve endings provide intense sexual pleasure, and all you need to do is gently separate the vaginal lips to find it.

Slide into the vaginal cavity to the clitoris, slide the tip of your thumb or index finger of one hand from the vaginal cavity up to and including the clitoris. With the other hand, hold the lips apart to expose the clitoris. You can also stimulate the clitoris by applying light pressure with your thumb in quick movements, creating a vibrating sensation alternating with drum-like taps.

During stimulation, alternate circular movements with the tip of your index finger on the clitoris, as if drawing small circles. This will add variety and intensity to the sensation, enriching the sensory experience.

Gently gather the hood of the clitoris between your thumb and forefinger, applying light pressure and gently rubbing between the two fingers. This can increase the sensitivity and effectiveness of the stimulation.

The clitoral area and especially its hood are extremely sensitive for many women. Gentle stimulation of this area can elicit powerful orgasms. Suggesting that she relax and breathe deeply during this phase can make subsequent experiences even more pleasurable, intense and beneficial.

After stimulating the clitoris, you can proceed to gently massage the vaginal cavity. Gently insert your middle finger inside and explore the cavity with slow and careful movements, varying depth and speed without interruption. Start from the opening of the vulva and, after having oiled your hands well with natural oil, insert your middle finger for about two centimeters, performing delicate circular movements both clockwise and counterclockwise. After at least two minutes of this type of massage, push your middle finger deeper and continue with circular movements, alternating between in and out, up and down, always keeping the palm of your hand facing upwards.

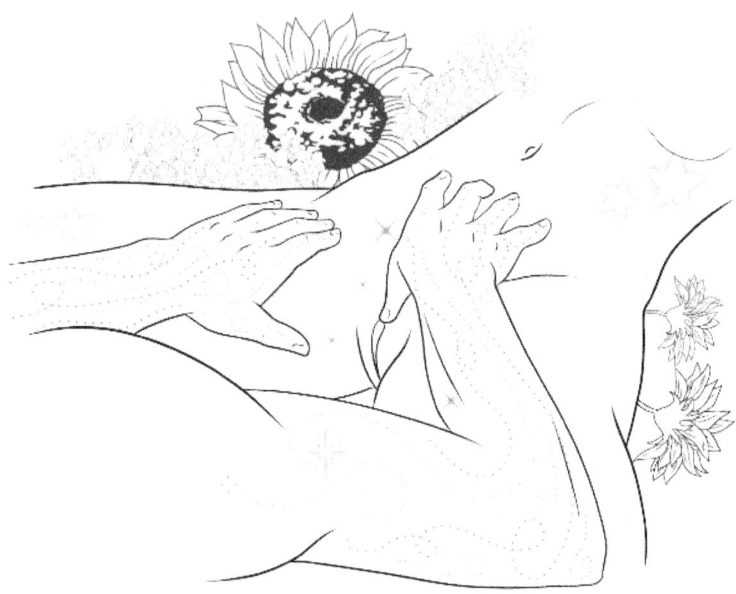

*Vibration of the thumb on the clitoris with the addition of a continuous pressure.*

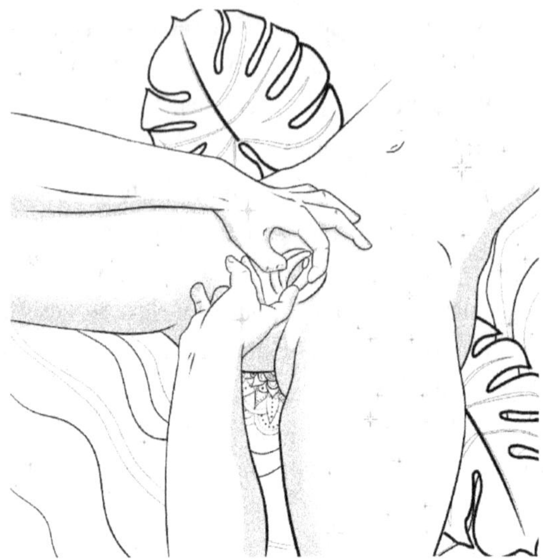

*Sliding massage with the finger, from the cavity to the clitoris and vice versa.*

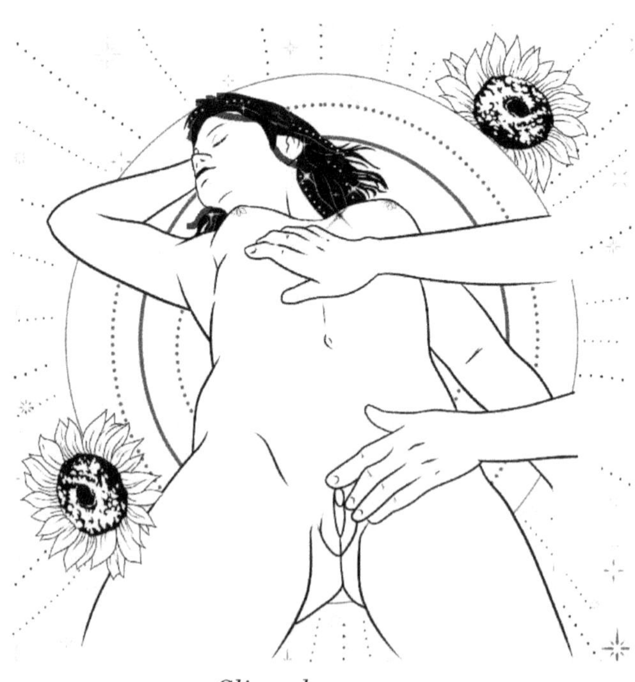

*Clitoral massage.*

# Massage of the G-Spot

Now you can start massaging the "G" spot, keeping yourself inside the vaginal cavity, place your middle finger just beyond the pubic bone, with the palm facing upwards. This area has a different consistency, more spongy. It is the famous "G" spot in tantric practice, the sacred point as seen previously. To stimulate it, slightly bend your middle finger to increase the pressure on the point and start performing delicate circular movements.

After massaging with a slow and constant rhythm for a few minutes, you can vary the pressure, speed and movement of your fingers. In addition to the middle finger, you can also introduce your index finger inside the Yoni, maintaining the same type of stimulation.

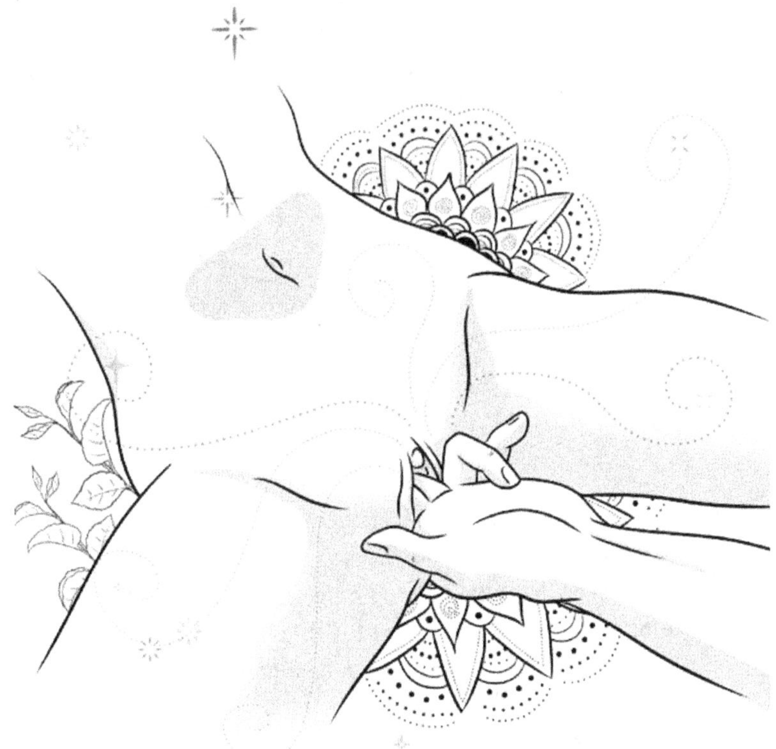

*Massage of the G-spot.*

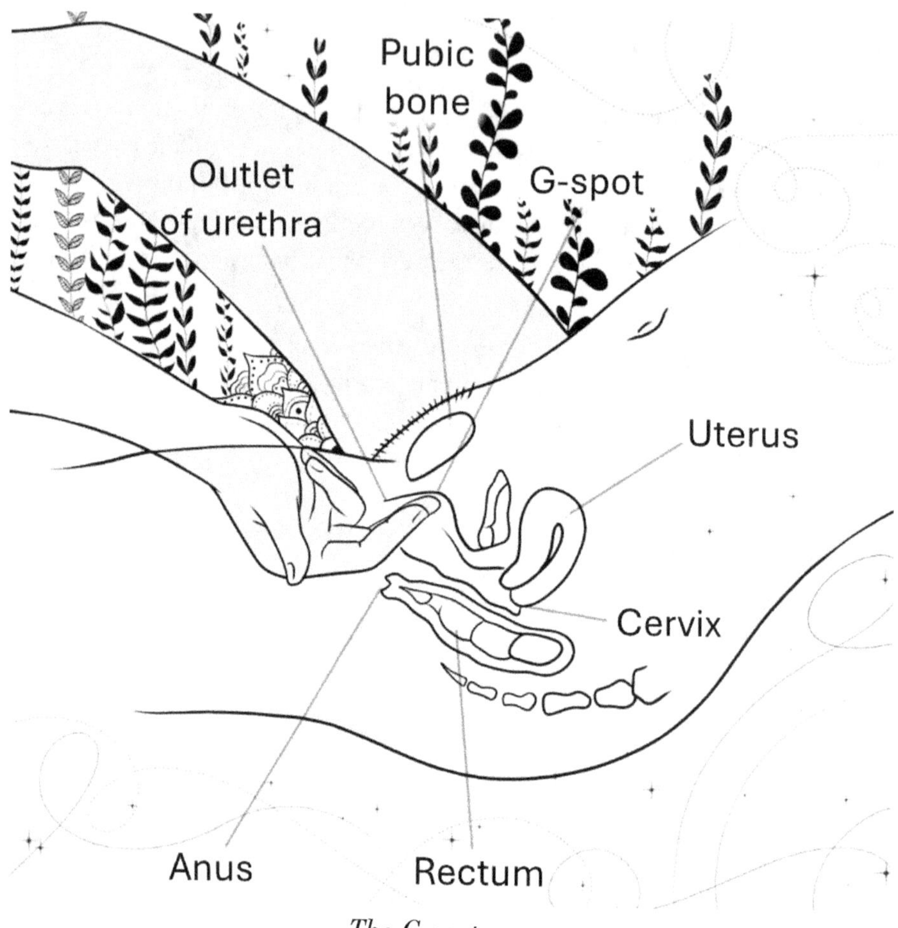


*The G-spot map.*

You can vary the stimulation by gently inserting your fingers in and out of the vaginal cavity. If you continue with this type of massage for several minutes, you will be able to access the deepest emotions of the woman, thus bringing her to an intense orgasm. Regarding the movement of fingers inside Yoni, here are some other techniques to enhance the effect of the massage and maintain variety:

- Stimulate the G-spot with your middle finger in a rhythmic way, pressing and releasing it as if you were playing a drum, maintaining gentle pressure.
- Occasionally massage the abdomen, chest, and breast while stimulating the G-spot to spread pleasure throughout the body. This type of massage can lead to the experimentation of multiple orgasms.

- As Yoni opens, you can insert your index finger and also the ring finger along with the middle, keeping the fingers slightly flexed for fluid movements in and out of the vaginal cavity.
- Simultaneously stimulate the G-spot and the clitoris, to lead her to the experience of a mixed orgasm, combining the clitoral and vaginal ones. According to Tantra, this is considered one of the greatest mysteries of the universe! If the receiver agrees, gently insert your little finger into the anus while you stimulate the clitoris with circular or swinging movements with the other hand.

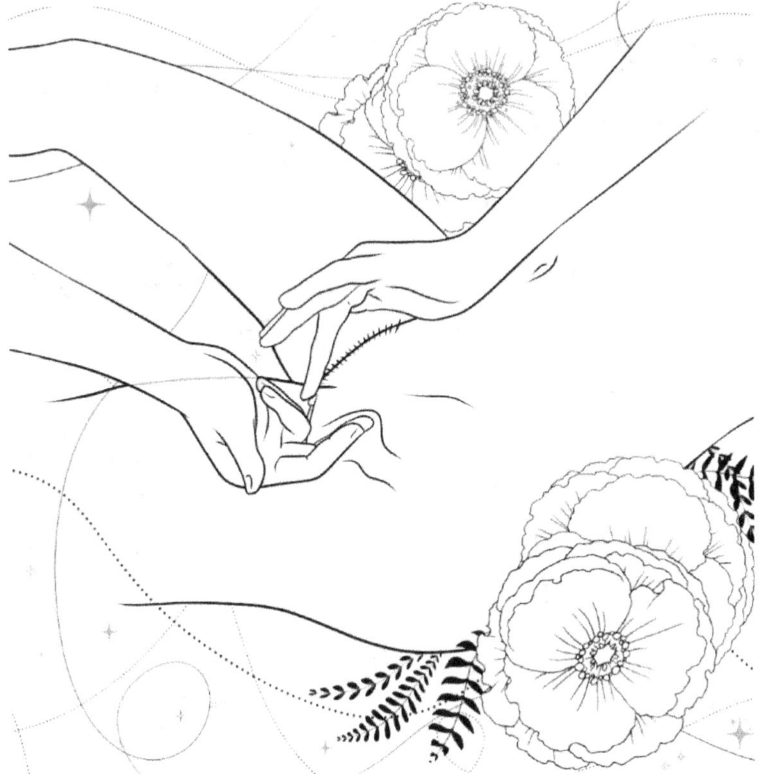

*Simultaneous stimulation of the G-spot and clitoris.*

The stimulation of the G-spot likely causes the woman an urgent need to urinate, which could be the urge to ejaculate. Since she can ejaculate before or after orgasm with a flow coming out of the urethra, when she feels this stimulus, it is important that she relaxes as much as possible and that she lets it simply go.

## Uterine Massage

Now, you are completely able to make a great massage in the vagina and cervix. A gentle and complete treatment of the vaginal region is essential for the well-being and pleasure of the woman. It is advisable to stimulate not only the G-spot but also the surrounding areas inside the vagina, still using your middle and index finger. You can also vary the pressure and speed by moving your wrist in different directions. To the right to involve the right side, to the left side downwards making circular movements with the middle and index fingers, and to the right at the bottom you can treat the cervix.

It is important to maintain a sensitivity and emotional connection during the entire procedure, exploring it all with care and love. After a few minutes, you will notice the way the woman reacts with pleasure and joy. Learning to master this massage can bring balance and well-being to your partner, offering serenity and harmony that may not be found elsewhere in life!

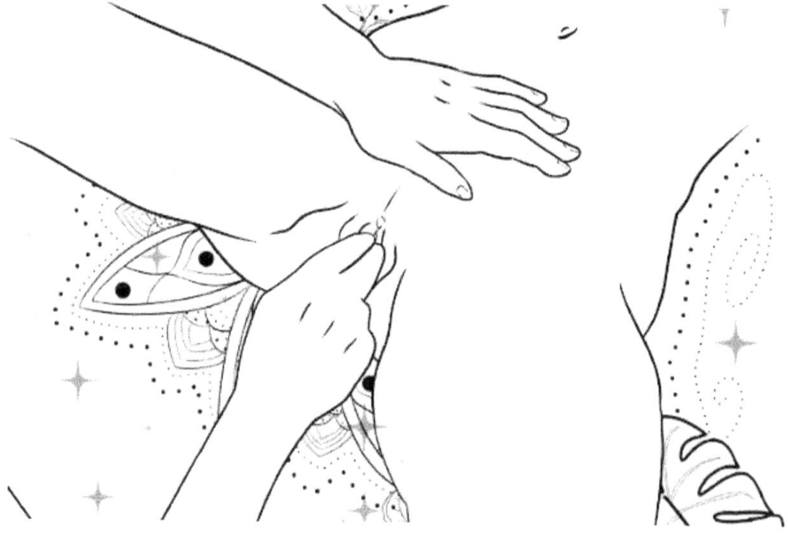

*Deep massage.*

Yoni massage does not have a set time since it does not necessarily end with the first orgasm, as others may follow. So, you can decide to end it when you want to or when the woman receiving the massage feels that it is time to stop, as she feels satisfied enough.

To vary the classic Yoni massage, you can change the angle or massage other areas of the vulva, also using more fingers. When the woman is completely satisfied and wants to stop, you can gently pull back your hand and cover it with a blanket, allowing her to relax and internalize the experience. It is important to stay close to her after the massage, transmitting tenderness and making her understand that it is a sensual and sweet experience and not just a mechanical one.

If you are a beginner, you may feel a little awkward at first, but over time, you will improve and know how to give more and more pleasure to your partner. It's normal to have some uncertainty about the points to touch, but with calm and delicacy, you will be able to identify those that give her more pleasure, becoming better and better every time.

This approach will enrich your relationship, bringing mutual pleasure and well-being, especially in such a hectic world where we live. Exploring new spheres of pleasure can contribute to a more fulfilling and radiant life as a couple!

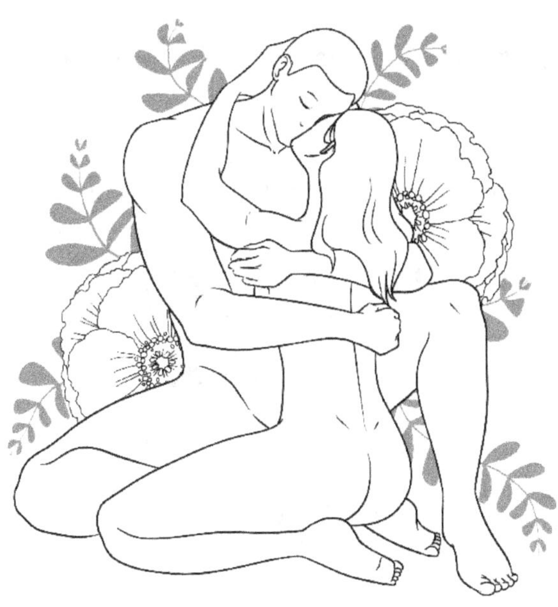

# Bonus: Download the Best Soundtrack to Use as Background During Your Massage

To download your digital Bonus, with the best music track for your Tantra and Yoni massage background, visit:

https://drive.google.com/drive/folders/115XCAGveJxLP2BN9UaOtRN0l-ZTA_j3DK?usp=sharing

or simply scan the QR code to directly download the file:

**Let the music overwhelm you and make the experience even more magical!**

# Conclusions

The tantric massage is an ancient and profound kind of art that lets us fully connect to our partner in an authentic way, awakening and balancing our inner energies. Nowadays, since prejudices and guilt can often withstand our true sense of being, Tantra can truly help us feel free from any chain holding us and present a new, different way to a major sense of awareness and well-being.

In this book, we have browsed through the tantric massage's main principles and foundations, for us to have a full guide to go to whenever we need to put it into practice, autonomously. We have tackled both theoretical and practical aspects, learning how Kundalini's awakening in us can forever change our lives, digging in often overlooked, practical details to apply this knowledge in a secure and competent way.

We have grappled with several ways to harmonize our seven chakras through prana, to guarantee the flowing of vital energy, as well as the perfect massage environment preparation, through an integration of the four elements and the five senses. Also, we have studied more about the importance of breathing and meditation as preparative acts to Yoni, discovering the vulvar sacred anatomy and the most suitable massage techniques for this area.

Now, it is up to your commitment and understanding to put what you have learned into practice. If you manage to, you will be able to offer the very best, transformative experience to your beloved, to bring physical, emotional, and spiritual wellness.

I truly hope this reading can be a gateway to the holistic world for you and that it may inspire you to keep on learning more about tantra and its related practices. The tantric massage not only represents a cure for the body but also for the soul. See this book as a personal and spiritual growth journey, leading you to the discovery of new well-being dimensions and a deeper kind of connection.

I wish that all this knowledge may be with you every day and enrich your being even more, letting you live a fuller, mindful, and harmonious life.

If the information here has helped you and you are willing to keep on receiving more suggestions about the holistic world, we invite you to review your experience and share what you have learned!

Your opinion matters to us and it will surely help us to grant you an even better service in the future.

Thank you for choosing us!

If you need a treatment and/or have any suggestions and/or questions about the related content, or if you simply want an insight, you can reach out to:

htmperinfo@gmail.com

If you want to continue to go deeper into the holistic and Tantric world, we invite you to follow us on social media:

**@holistictantramassages**

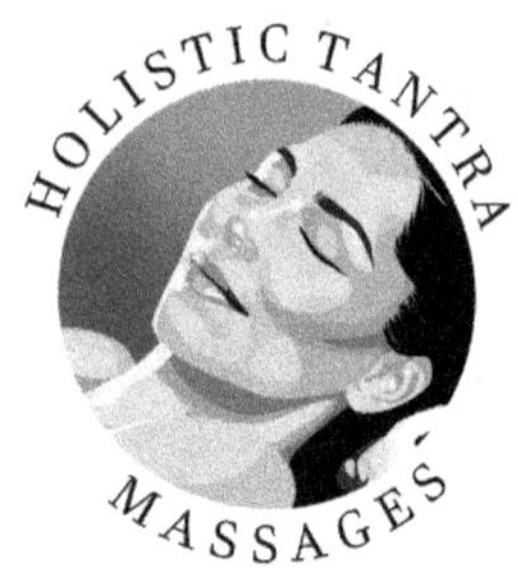